It Takes 2

Surviving Breast Cancer:
A Spouse's Story

By **Mark Brodinsky**

Dedication

This book is dedicated to every breast cancer survivor and to all those who have yet to fight, but will face their own journey and hope to win. It's also dedicated to the memory of my father-in-law, Debbie's dad, Jerry Gross, who lost his battle against cancer and left us much too soon. We miss you, Dad, and live to honor your memory.

Acknowledgements

THE ROMAN POET Horace says, "Adversity has the effect of eliciting talents, which, in prosperous times, would have lain dormant." If not for Debbie, her illness, her fight, her courage, and her inspiration, I never would have gone back to my roots to write, to share emotion, love, and perspective in a way which has transformed me and apparently others who have been touched by our story.

I thank my wife for being the incredible woman she is and our friends who supported and brought peace and comfort to our lives throughout our journey. We are forever in your debt.

I also thank our two miracles, our daughters Sophie and Emily, for being the loving and supportive wind beneath our wings. Girls, we love you to the moon and back.

And I need to acknowledge the Dream Team who helped make this book a reality, led by my assistant, Lisa Norris. I also want to thank Holly Burke for her incredible cover art and to Patti McKenna, my very first editor. You never forget your first. And there are many more of you, so many I would need to write another book just to include all the "thank yous."

Another book? ... Hmmm ... maybe I will.

Mark

Book cover design by Holly Burke

Back cover photo by Adam Oberfeld

Printed in the United States of America

Contents

Foreword

THE GIFT OF authoring this foreword was bestowed upon me not long after my baby sister, Debbie, was the subject of an incredibly important celebration. She was one year cancer free. A year prior, I sat on the bathroom floor at Mercy Hospital, offering just about anything for Debbie to survive her double-mastectomy surgery and make a complete recovery. I learned only recently, in reflecting upon the journal entries that form the foundation of this work, that her husband, my brother-in-law and dear friend of many years, spent that morning in a similar way.

Funny, I've known Mark for two decades now. He was the friend of a high school boyfriend and, for sure, the prize in that CrackerJack box! For all these years, Mark and I have been there for each other through unspeakable joy, and seemingly unbearable pain. From sharing the simple pleasures of baseball on a summer night (though I know he takes issue with my waning love for baseball over the years), to the indescribable glee of hearing the words "it's a girl!" four blessed times over (and occasionally questioning that glee as we raise our four 'tweens and teenagers). From the disappointment of a missed field goal during Ravens post-season play, to the gut-wrenching torture of my father's cancer diagnosis, followed by his cruel and untimely death.

Ironically, Mark has teased me many times over in those decades for being too overprotective of Debbie. "Mother Teresa" I was dubbed, as the two of them artfully avoided telling me of the white water rafting "incident" from which Debbie now proudly wears a badge of honor on her shin. Heck, they probably played Rock-Paper-Scissors when debating who would have to relay the news about the ATV ride gone bad for Debbie, leaving a broken wrist behind. Of course, these came after years of "oopses" and "how did that happens"—all of which inevitably made my sister the pillar of strength she is today. She is unspeakably amazing, beautiful-inside-and-out, and an indestructible force.

Reflecting back on May 10, 2012, I sat on that bathroom floor looking the beast in the eyes of my family for now the third time, first with my mother, then with my father, and now with my baby sister. I recall asking, "How can I manage this again?" Strangely, in hindsight, the only thing I had to manage was me. You see, after about 40 years of worry—and, as I've suggested, there were countless reasons worthy of worry—I just sat by, rather awestruck, as I watched my brother-in-law do it all. Not only did Mark provide care—the best care—to meet my unspoken, yet otherwise insurmountable, standards, he also articulated the words that I—and many of us who love Debbie beyond words—could not. It was through Mark's candor and brutal honesty that we, too, could find release.

Now, with that same brand of authenticity, Mark shares his gift of writing, with a passion and zeal we should all be fortunate enough to possess. Try, as I will, to let these traits infect you as you read. May Mark's talent and Debbie's fortitude be resources from which we all may draw.

Alisa Cummins

Preface

BEFORE I MADE the decision to publish, I read a book by Guy Kawasaki, *APE: Author, Publisher, Entrepreneur – How to Publish a Book*. In his guide on self-publishing, Kawasaki states, "If you thought starting a book was hard, wait until you try to finish one." Truer words have rarely been written. At the time of writing this preface, there are only two weeks to go before the date I want the first physical copy of *It Takes 2* printed and in my hands. I made the announcement on the date, I put the flag in the sand, and we are not yet complete with book layout, cover art, table of contents, bio, back cover, or last minute revisions. When I finally hold a copy of the book, I will be amazed it was completed and on time. Yet, I have no doubt it will. Have the vision, develop a plan, strive for the goal. It's a whole new world in my life, exhausting, exhilarating, frustrating and life affirming ... all at the same time.

Yet the process pales in comparison to what my wife Debbie has faced since April of 2012. It is her journey, our journey, that keeps life in perspective and why I will never again look at any problem as insurmountable. With her courage, spirit of survival, and grace under pressure, Debbie set the bar so high I can live the rest of my life and barely come close. My wife is a wonder to behold, and I'm the lucky one, I get to hold her close.

I purposely kept Debbie out of the loop during much of what needed to take place to make this book happen. One, I didn't want her to relive the experience, even while she is still going through it, and secondly, I'm not convinced she was convinced I would get it done. The last thing I would ever want to do is disappoint her, especially after all she has endured.

But I can tell you with all sincerity there is nothing I wanted more since the day Debbie reached the milestone of being one year cancer free than to complete and publish the book you now hold in your hands or read on your tablet.

This is my gift to my love, a way to give back, to share our story, and honor my wife for her sacrifice that saved our family. From the day I decided to write the first word, the journal, this book, was a labor of love, and it's part of a dream fulfilled to publish Debbie's story, our story, to stand for all time.

It is my hope you find your time well spent in the pages ahead. As you read, I ask you to share my heart and you, too, may stand in awe of the woman I am honored to call my wife.

From my heart to yours, thanks for caring.

Mark

Introduction

Speak from the heart, and everyone who has one will buy in. That's what I have done for the past year, as my wife, Debbie, a beautiful 40-year-old woman, mother of our two young daughters, battled the beast ... breast cancer. I did my best to document the journey and offer my perspective, my insight, and most important, to offer my support, love, and devotion throughout the journey. Along the way, I have learned that my g.a.l., gratitude, appreciation, and love, might be the strongest three words on the planet.

These are the three words that come from the heart, the ones I have tried to put on display as I have stood by my wife's side during this past year. They say three is a magic number, and these three words are at the very center, the very foundation of our lives. Tap into their message and you can experience wonderful, magical events, maybe even a miracle or two. We did. Tune them out and you will be lost in the whirlwind that is the journey of life. It is not hard to get lost.

This is the story of a journey inside our journey. You might say it is never ending, I might say you are right. This story is meant to be one of inspiration, education, hope, and love. We lived it, or should I say we are *living it*, because there really is no finish line. The physical healing has happened; the emotional healing may forever be a work in progress. But such is life, yours, mine, ours. It just so happens we had a visitor come crash the party of our lives, breast cancer.

Breast cancer. The words resonate when they are spoken, every time they are spoken. They carry with them a stigma of concern, of dread, of fear, and of loss. It just might be the most unfair cancer on this earth. Sure, for anyone who has cancer, it's unfair. But just because you are a woman and you have breasts, why should you as a gender be more at risk, more afflicted? It's almost as if G-d is trying to even the score. Because you can give life, He chooses to present you with the challenge, as a woman, of fighting for yours.

The statistics are still numbing. Breast cancer is the most common cancer among American women, except for skin cancers. About 1-in-8 women in the U.S. will develop invasive breast cancer during her lifetime. The American Cancer Society's most recent predictions for 2013:

- About 232,340 new cases of invasive breast cancer will be diagnosed in women.

- About 64,640 new cases of carcinoma in situ (CIS) will be diagnosed (CIS is non-invasive and is the earliest form of breast cancer).

- About 39,620 women will die from breast cancer.

One death is too many. How and why can something so special, so unique, so beautiful, not only in shape and size, but in the ability to sustain life after birth ... how is it they become the conduit for such pain and suffering?

To be completely transparent, we got lucky. Actually, luck had very little to do with it. Luck is made when preparation meets opportunity. Somehow, someway, despite the shock of it all, my wife was prepared to face the challenge head-on with a decision that would change her life and ours forever. It is her courage which led us down the path to what you might call good luck. Good luck, because as of this writing, she is healed and cancer free. However, you don't reach that moment without great sacrifice; as with any victory, there is a price to pay. It's as if someone upstairs has decided that nothing worthwhile in life, nothing worth fighting for, should come gift-wrapped. The gift must be the result of a great battle. Debbie, my wife, fought the fight of her life, and won. We, myself, my daughters, our family, our friends, our social media network, and countless other co-workers and acquaintances could only watch in wonder at the focus and fortitude of the woman I am blessed to call my wife.

For certain people, being presented with the challenge of cancer is a call to arms. For some, it is a reason to run and hide. For others, there is no time to fight because it is too late. Fortunately, the latter are becoming rarer in America as the number of breast cancer *survivors* grow.

So this, this is the story of a survivor, Debbie's story, told mostly through my eyes. Sometimes my eyes were red with anger because of the unfairness of it all; sometimes they were open wide in wonder as I gained insight into the illness, the process, and the lessons learned from my wife and how she handled herself. And sometimes my eyes were squinting through the tears of sadness, fear, and even despair. This is Debbie's story. This is My story. This is Our story. This is the story of a journey through breast cancer and its greatest lesson: that gratitude, appreciation, and love can have an effect, an effect on healing, on hearts, on minds, and can even help create a miracle or two. This journal is my gift to Debbie, to myself, to you.

Breast Cancer: A love story. Let's begin.

1 From Sea to Shocking "C"

IT WAS NEVER going to happen. Cancer is something that affects other people, but it's not going to happen to us, no way, not inside the four walls of our home. We had been through enough. My wife, Debbie, had been through enough. Her mom, Sharon, is a 20-year plus breast cancer survivor. Just 2 and 1/2 years earlier, we lost Debbie's father to esophageal cancer. We stood by his hospital bed, in shock and despair as they turned off the machines, and then we watched him slip away. Her dad, my buddy and one of my favorite people, was diagnosed in June 2009. By November he was gone. He got an infection following surgery to remove the cancer, and he never recovered. Yes, enough was enough.

Now, it was April 2012. Just days before our world turned upside down, we stepped off the cruise ship after an unbelievable vacation with my family, my sister-in-law, brother-in-law, my nieces, and my mother-in-law, who had treated us to the trip. Yes, life was good, or at least it was on solid ground. But we had a date coming up that week to check out an irregularity in Debbie's right breast, one the doctors kept telling us was nothing. After a great vacation like the one we had just finished, all the good karma was in our favor. Or so we thought.

"It Looks Benign to Me"
(Before Diagnosis)
Written April 10, 2012 10:13 p.m.

"They can't stop the bleeding." "I feel faint." "There's a lot of blood."

These are the texts I am getting from Debbie, while I sit with my mother-in-law in the waiting room at Northwest Hospital. Wasn't it supposed to be a needle-guided MRI biopsy? Why was Debbie bleeding? And why couldn't they get it to stop? Should we call a doctor? Oh, they are already back there, doing a real bang-up job. Sounds like all is well.

It wasn't much fun waiting and wondering what was really happening. Apparently, the needle-guided biopsy had been finished, but the numbing agent "causes some people to bleed excessively" is what the radiologist told us, the same one who gave my mother-in-law and me his extensive credentials before he gave us what he believed to be the results.

The MRI had been arranged after a mammogram in March showed an irregularity in Debbie's right breast, and then the ultrasound, which had shown nothing. Debbie's breasts were cystic and dense to begin with, so the only way to know for sure what was going on was to go in and take a sample of the irregular tissue. Apparently, what we didn't know in advance is when they take the sample out, they insert a marker to easily identify the spot the next time there is a mammogram—except the marker didn't take, so the team had to go back in to do it again. The radiologist later told us this was the first time in 25 years this had happened to him. Zip-a-dee-doo-da day.

When our "guy" came out to tell us what he believed to be his "diagnosis at a glance" of the tissue cells removed, he was fairly confident. "I would say there's only a 1-in-10 chance the tissue sample is malignant. I've been doing this for a long time, and it looks benign to me."

The appointment was twice as long as it should have been because of the team of "experts" going back in to remark the spot where they removed the tissue sample, after the first marker failed. It was taking forever, and they hadn't really stopped the bleeding completely. Debbie was being medically beaten-up. Her breast looks like a fighter's face after going 15 rounds. She has bruised terribly and developed a hematoma from all the trauma that site has suffered.

Still, the medical professional, in his professional opinion, has provided us hope. He said there is only a 1-in-10 chance it's malignant. I heard him, and I keep repeating that sentence over and over in my head. We wait for the pathology results, but the message we left the hospital with seems to be positive.

Now it's time to rest, ice the area where they plunged the needle into her breast, and "chill" until we get word from the lab. Debbie is sleeping uncomfortably, in pain and badly bruised from the biopsy. We won't know for a few days what the test of the tissue sample will show. So, for now, the show must go on.

Thanks for caring,

Mark

Forever Changed
Written April 13, 2012 10:10 p.m.

I don't remember what she said; I just remember where I was.

Friday the 13th, April 2012. This is a day we will never forget. I'm at my car, parked just outside the bank on this beautiful Friday morning. I had just popped the trunk for some reason and was standing outside looking in when the cell phone rang. It was Debbie. And she was sad.

Sad is an understatement. I could hear it through her tears, a garbled, quick explanation that the radiologist had called, and it wasn't benign, it was malignant, or maybe she used the word cancer. I honestly don't remember. All I knew was Debbie was at work, and I was miles away. I couldn't get to her at that moment. I couldn't hold her—all I could do was listen to her fear and pain through the phone and through those tears. I felt like I was standing in quicksand. I hopped back in the car, because it was windy and I couldn't hear all of what Debbie was saying. She said the radiologist called her at work and said he wanted to talk to her... then he asked if she was sitting down! She knew then it was not going to be a great moment. He said the pathology report showed a malignancy inside her nipple duct, cancer in-situ, but the concern was the invasive tumor outside the duct, that was a bigger issue. Then I heard the phone cut out.

It was Debbie's call-waiting. Someone was calling in, either her mom, or her sister, or a good friend. I don't know, I don't remember, but Debbie wanted to take the call. She said she would call me right back. Sure, just like any other day. Except today wasn't like any other day, neither will be the days to come, I'm sure. Life has done what life does—throws down the gauntlet and then looks you straight in the eye and asks, "Okay, what are you going to do now?"

I'll tell you what I was going to do—I was going to get to Debbie. So I started driving. Where was I going? I wasn't sure. Deb was a good 30 miles away at work, and was she staying, or going? Was I going home? What about my two daughters? What about my mother-in-law, a breast cancer survivor herself, what was she thinking? What about my sister-in-law? What was going on? What was the next move? I wasn't sure at that moment; I was just sure I was driving.

Then the phone rang. Debbie was calling back.

The journey of a thousand miles begins with one small step. The wheels were in motion. Debbie said her sister, Alisa, was already making calls to doctors. Alisa, G-d bless her, when a crisis strikes, is all over it. She takes charge, and her baby sister had just been diagnosed with breast cancer, so she wasn't messing around. Neither was their mom, Sharon. My mother-in-law's boyfriend, Lloyd, has a connection, and, through that connection, we have a shot at getting in to see one of the best breast cancer surgeons in Baltimore.

I now had an answer as to my destination. I had not dared make a single call, for fear of missing Debbie's next one. She was leaving work, and we would meet up at a restaurant near our home. A couple of close friends were headed there, as well. I needed to see Debbie, and they wanted to see her, too. In just those few minutes after the call today that started it all, the outpouring of support and love was already in full swing.

Debbie and I pulled up in the parking lot at almost the same time. I got out and went around to her car, and we embraced. Deb had calmed down since the phone call, maybe reassured that steps were already being taken to get in to see a doctor and discuss what was going to happen next. It felt good to hold her for even a moment, and, in that moment, I knew it was somehow going to be okay, although not sure exactly how, or why, but we will be victorious in the end.

Love is the most powerful healing force in the world. It's like a drug, like medicine for the soul, and this love is going to make a difference in whatever is going to come next. We will not be defeated. Life will go on. My wife, my daughters, will be okay. This story will have a very different ending than the one that had been written just three years earlier when we lost Debbie's dad to cancer. I know it with every part of my being. We are going to win.

Thanks for caring,

Mark

Guestbook Entries

Deb! You have our love and support. Mark! You two have our love and support! Brodinsky kids, you ladies rock. But seriously, Frank and I cannot express how blessed we are to have met two wonderful people in our lives. We love you both and will support you and anyone else that needs a smile, hug, laugh, or just to feel grounded.

Love, Frank Chiovaro +Daisy Kim

Just signed on here to let you know how very much we all love you, Debra Lyn.

As I've mentioned in the past, you are one of the strongest women I know and you are my hero. You have made it through so many difficult times and you will make it through this one as well. You have so many people who love you and are here for you anytime, day or night.

Love you, Sherri Thomas

Deb, you are truly one of my favorite people in the whole world! I have known you for most of my life and love every minute I get to spend with you. I can't imagine how scary all of this is for you but I do know that you are an amazing woman with an amazing support system and that love, with your strength, will get you through this. You all will be in my thoughts and prayers and I'm here if you need anything. Love you.

Susan Stepke

Debbie's Decision: A Life Transformed

Written April 19, 2012 9:01pm

Six days after diagnosis, there we were today, me, Debbie, her mom, Sharon, and her sister, Alisa, sitting in the office staring at the breast surgeon. Two weeks earlier, before this all began, we were just leaving the ship after a great cruise with the family. Now we are sailing in a different direction and in rough seas. Scary to say the least.

Debbie and I were sitting at the desk, watching Dr. Friedman from the Mercy Breast Center as he looked intently at the films from the MRI needle-guided biopsy. Dr. Friedman then drew some pictures for us, showing us the tumor in the right nipple duct and the invasive tumor just outside of that duct. That's the real area of concern. Yes, she... we... have cancer. So what now?

Debbie has made her decision. But she didn't want to make it official, or officially public, until Dr. Friedman went over the options today. He is recommending a lumpectomy. The tumor is not that large, they could go in, cut it out, test the lymph nodes, and then we would see about post-treatment, chemotherapy, radiation, etc. Of course, that doesn't mean the cancer wouldn't, or couldn't, come back or surface somewhere else. All we can be sure of is no one can be sure. How comforting.

My wife was having none of this. Deb was pretty matter of fact. She told the good doctor she wanted to have a double mastectomy, both breasts removed... for good. Even writing this on my laptop now, with my wife sleeping by my side, it's hard to go back and relive that moment today. I can still picture Dr. Friedman looking back at Debbie from across his desk. He definitely paused for a second when she said it. I truly believe, just for a moment, even he was caught off guard how sure Debbie was about her decision.

It is a choice that she, I, and everyone knows will change her life... our lives ... forever.

Yet, it has to be done. Although I hate to see it happen, I understand. There is family history; there are our two daughters to think about. Debbie doesn't want to keep looking over her shoulder, keep fearing every mammogram and every test. And with the bi-lateral mastectomy, there will be, as long as there is nothing in the lymph nodes, a greater certainty that cancer would be gone. Forever.

Even at this moment, it still hurts my heart to relive today. Hurts my head to think about it. Hurts my soul to appreciate the sacrifice Debbie is making to save us. Love makes you do crazy things; it also makes you do the right thing when your back is up against the wall, to protect those you love. Debbie's decision shows the greatest love of all.

Everybody wants to meet a hero. I'm lucky, I'm married to one.

Thanks for caring,

Mark

Guestbook Entries:

Deb

I'm a 28-year survivor of the same kind of breast cancer. Keep your spirits high, know that you'll be there for your husband and children. Praying for a healthy journey for you.
Fondly, Carleen Basso

We have known and loved Deb since her birth and have cherished her soft heart and her strength. What we so appreciate is Mark's ability to express his love and support because we know that she will be able to rely upon it and upon him. No words can really capture our distress that all of you have to go through this. We keep you in our hearts and our prayers.

Gail Kass

I want to tell you what an incredible role model you are to your daughters, your friends... and me. You show me that it will all be fine, more than fine... it will be better. You show me that it's okay to take it slowly, make your decisions, get your affairs in order and then get ready to win the fight. You have prepared yourself to battle. You won't need to, you have won. You just need to get across the finish line. We will all be with you when you cross, smiling, cheering, and maybe tears. Tears of joy because we knew all along you would be fine and tears because you did it. It will be over before you know it, and YOU WILL look back and say to yourself, "How did I ever do this?"

Due to the love and support of your loving husband, your precious family, caring friends, and your constant desire to heal and be rid of this disease.... YOU WILL SMILE WITH PRIDE AND LAUGHTER. WE WILL BE SMILING WITH YOU, ALWAYS.

Love,

Gina Millstein

Breaking News
Written April 20th, 2012 9:30 p.m.

Time for a special report. We just learned this evening that the mastectomy and the reconstructive surgery will be scheduled for Thursday, May 10th at Mercy Hospital. Dr. Bernard

Chang from Mercy will perform the reconstructive surgery and handle the implants. In the end, this will be okay and Debbie will be one of the survivors. I know it.

Never thought we would be going through anything like this... but who does? It is simply another avenue on the journey of life. Country singer Gary Allan has a song, "Life Ain't Always Beautiful." But my wife is, my girls are, our family is, our incredible friends are... and that's what it's all about. With all your love and support, how can we lose? Debbie will need all of it as she begins the next chapter of her life... and our lives together. Already we need to say thanks to so many for reaching out and letting us know you are there. It is a true blessing.

My wife is a fighter. No doubt about that. She will come out of this on the other side, better than she went in. The struggle of life does not beat you, it only makes you stronger. I am married to the most beautiful, funny, smart incredible woman... who also just happens to be an outstanding mother to my two girls. No cancer is going to take that away, and it will not defeat us.

Deb gets her strength from our girls, Sophie and Emily, from her sister, Alisa, and maybe most of all from her mom and my mother-in-law, Sharon, who herself is a 20-year-breast-cancer-survivor. She is leading by example. You fight back, you don't get beat, you ride the emotional rollercoaster, and when the ride ends, you get up and look back and realize you were scared, but you made it. That's all that matters.

"The journey of a thousand miles must begin with a single step. To know the road ahead, ask those coming back."

Those who have made the journey before Debbie give us strength.

Those who love us give us hope and light.

Those we have never met, but are living the same challenge... you have our support.

Thanks for being there. We couldn't ask for more.

And thanks for caring,

Mark

Waiting

Written April 22, 2012 7:17 a.m.

It's been several days now since we set up our Caringbridge webpage.

Thanks to those who are visiting. My hope is you will take a moment now and then to share a positive thought with Debbie. The physicality of what will take place is easier explained, defined, and documented with science and medicine. The emotional toll is impossible for any of us, even the survivors (because each story and person is different), to clearly define. I believe it is a mix of fear, hope, anger, and love, but how do all the pieces fit together?

The bottom line is I just want my wife to be well, physically and emotionally. With that end in mind, here's a thought:

> "Hope is like the sun, which, as we journey toward it, casts the shadow of our burden behind us."
> —Samuel Smiles

Looking forward to putting this all behind us.

Thanks for caring,

Mark

The Week Ahead

Written April 23, 2012 8:38 a.m.

The week ahead will bring more waiting, booking a pre-op physical, and at the end of the week, we will meet with the other VIP in this procedure: Dr. Bernard Chang at Mercy Hospital. Dr. Chang is the Director of Plastic and Reconstructive Surgery and will explain the steps involved in the reconstruction and breast implants to be used once the double mastectomy is complete.

Debbie is doing "okay." She is strong, resilient—but I know how sad she is—sad about what has happened, sad about what she has to face, sad she will miss out on some important events, including Asia Gorman's Bat Mitzvah, which is just two days after the surgery. For those who don't know, the Gorman's are like family to us. Not just like—they are. I know it pains Debbie not to be able to be there, but this surgery has to happen now, and the goal is to make sure Deb is there for EVERY other occasion to come. We love you, Gorman family.

Last night, as we watched a program on a high-profile couple dealing with the same challenge, I told Debbie that when it first happens, your initial thought is "my wife has cancer." As the days progress, you realize your partnership means we are both dealing with the same issue, at least emotionally. I just wish I could take the pain away for her. While I know the final result will be life moving forward, the journey to that destination will change us both.

> "Though no one can go back and make a brand new start, anyone can start from now and make a brand new ending." —Carl Bard

Thanks for caring,

Mark

The Latest

Written April 27, 2012 6:56 p.m.

Less than two weeks to go. The journey continues... and today, the next stop on the rollercoaster ride.

Today, we visited with Dr. Bernard Chang from the Mercy Breast Center. There are two sides to this. My wife (besides being incredibly beautiful) is simply the strongest person I know. She has made her decision to go with a bi-lateral mastectomy and has not wavered. After watching the 10-minute pre-appointment DVD about the "reconstruction," I was ready to leave. It was making me sick to my stomach, but Debbie watched it and was unwavering in her decision.

Don't get me wrong; it's the best decision. But surgery is surgery, is surgery. There are risks, and there is recovery, and it's far from pretty, but with the right attitude and the incredible support we have already experienced, I have no doubt it will all be okay in the end. The end will bring a new beginning. Plenty of information was shared today, plenty of questions answered.

The big picture is clear, get Deb healthy and work out the details of the reconstruction over the next 10-12 months. I never knew the process could take that long, I never realized the scars never completely heal, I never knew how much I would hurt for her... never knew how angry I would be that Debbie has to resort to this decision. But who am I kidding... I always knew Debbie would make the right one, not for her, which is last in her mind, but the right decision to make sure she will always be here for the girls... and for me. Let's face it, I could never be the same person without her.

And so it goes. Another small step along the journey... there are more appointments to come before the "new beginning," before Debbie officially becomes a survivor. Although in reality, she already is.

Up next, the pre-op physical, then a meeting with the head nurse and occupational therapist at the Mercy Breast Center. It's all medicine, all scientific, all black and white. The colors in between are the emotions, the feelings, the fear, the hope, and the faith. All take their toll, all keep us on edge, yet all keep us moving forward to the end game, for Debbie to get well and be here. Forever.

> "Life is not about the breaths you take, but the moments that take your breath away."
>
> —George Strait

Thanks for caring,

Mark

10 Days

Written May 1st, 2012 9:48 a.m.

May 1st means we have 10 days to go. I know it's also a bittersweet birthday for my sister-in-law, Alisa. We love you, sis.

Update: The pre-op physical is out of the way, which consisted of a visit to the primary care doctor, blood work, and a chest x-ray, the results of which we should know in a few days. To our good friend, Jenny, thanks for being there today and taking Deb to her appointment.

Although Debbie doesn't talk about it too much, I think because it makes what was "surreal" seem all too real, Deb is so thankful for all the love and support she has been receiving. We can't say enough about all the cards, messages, and good wishes sent our way. It all means the world to us. With support like this, we can't lose. Not that there was ever a doubt. Every positive message and word of encouragement makes a difference. The battle will be won. We don't expect it to be easy, but we're ready. Attitude is everything, and we are positive this is the right decision, and when all is said and done, it will mean a long, happy life ahead.

10 days to go. 10 days to a new beginning. 10 days to freedom.

Thanks for caring,

Mark

Fun, Fear, and Hope
Written May 4, 2012 10:59 p.m.

With less than a week to go before surgery, Debbie and I got the chance to get away for a night, staying downtown at the Marriott Waterfront. (Thanks for the upgrade, Keith). We basically ate and drank our way through Fells Point on Thursday night. We had a blast, good to have the one-on-one time with a week to go before surgery. 15 years of marriage and we still enjoy every minute of our alone time together. I couldn't ask for more. We even went back in to Fells on Friday for lunch—before heading to Mercy Breast Center for three more important appointments Friday afternoon.

On the way to our next round of appointments, Deb was scared and tense. She was nauseous driving over to the hospital. How quickly 24 hours of fun turn back into fear and stress when you come back to reality and the somber feelings of the present situation.

The first appointment was with Marsha, the head nurse at the Mercy Breast Center. She was terrific. She was interested in everything about Debbie, including how she arrived at her decision about the double mastectomy. (Marsha is a cancer survivor, double mastectomy.) She went over the directions for the big morning, including where to go—the surgery will actually take place at the Mary Catherine Bunting Center at Mercy. Marsha said the surgery could take five hours plus, depending on if the doctors are running on time and time in between the breast removal (tough to say those words) and the reconstruction process. Maybe making it more real than ever was the "drain kit" she gave us to take home. These drains will be part of Debbie for a week to 10 days and need to be changed twice a day. Sleeping will be rough, only on the back, no side, no stomach, and propped up with pillows all around. She'll need help getting out of and back into bed to get set-up properly. But, amazingly, no bandages, no dressings to change, the sutures are actually under the skin, with plenty of surgical glue holding things together. The idea is that this way, we limit the risk of infection.

I have to say, at least for me, Marsha's explanation, calm demeanor, and allowing us to ask any questions we wanted, made me feel better about things. She had a positive attitude about it all—heck, she's lived it. Nice to hear this from a survivor. For the first time since the diagnosis, I really felt like I was going to break down, not out of sadness, but out of relief, that maybe, just maybe, this might not be as tough as we thought, for as long as we thought. I can only hope.

The next appointment was with an occupational therapist, who took measurements and went over, step-by-step, the exercises Debbie needs to do a few times each day to promote healing and muscle development. She needs to be religious about those to heal as fast as possible and get full movement back. The therapist, Rebecca, was also great.

The third appointment was a quick one, a fitting in the breast cancer shop for garments Debbie will wear during and after surgery. The shop has everything you need, and you can purchase products from there after surgery. They have everything for the breast cancer survivor, from the proper support bras to bathing suits. It is a place of dignity for those who are forced to suffer the indignity of a cancer-induced mastectomy.

The hardest part is watching my wife, one of the strongest people I know, maintain that strength, even when I know she doesn't want to. We were given a lot of information, almost too much to digest in one day. I can see it in Deb's eyes as she listens... there's understanding, but fear. Fear about what she will have to go through in a few days and fear, despite all the facts they throw at you, of the unknown.

You know what, though... the only emotion stronger than fear is hope. That's what you hold onto; that's what our friends and family give us. That's what matters. It's how you get through the tough times. No matter what, the sun will rise and set—no matter what happens in your life, or in the lives of others. Every day is a new day. There is always tomorrow. The only goal, and my personal goal, is to make every tomorrow better for Deb.

So as the days turn into hours, the hours turn into minutes, and those minutes to seconds before surgery, we keep the faith. Thanks to all those who are keeping the faith right along with us.

Thanks for caring,

Mark

Guestbook Entries:

First, Mark... you are an incredibly gifted writer. Thank you for allowing "us," the readers to understand your day at the hospital with Debbie. Thank you for letting us know that she is in the best possible place, with such devoted people taking care of her, and that you are both remembering that HOPE is everything.

I feel blessed to be able to be a part of this journey that you have to go through... all of you... your entire family. We will do whatever Debbie wants or needs.

Gina Millstein

Debbie,

You know, of all the thousands of people that have ever worked for me, only a few have I ever called friend. You are one of those people. You have been an inspiration since the first day we met. I have no doubt that you will beat this! It will have challenges, but I believe that God only gives us what we can handle and you will handle this with grace and dignity. It won't be easy but you have what it takes to beat this and get back to living your life with the same zest you do everything with. Amie and I will be thinking about you daily, and please don't hesitate to ask if we can do anything at all. When you are on the path to recovery, perhaps we will share a chocolate top together. I look forward to that day soon. Be brave, be strong and be ready for getting back to your normal life as soon as possible.

Alan Smith

Dearest Debbie-

One of the many things I admire about you is how you have survived so much hardship with grace, humor, and love. This journey you are on will end up being another accomplishment in survival. You are a survivor and will remain a survivor for many long years to come! I know it in my gut, as do all the people who love you.

Anything you need... anything at all, I am a hop skip and a jump away. I love you, girlie! Sending all good blessings your way...

Lori Vento

2 Days to Go

Written May 8, 2012 9:31 p.m.

How does that song go... "All you need is love"? Keep the positive messages coming. Keep the faith. Deb is anxious and afraid about what lies ahead on Thursday.

It's late, and we're tired, but for those who have been asking, tomorrow night I will post details about when, what, and how everything will happen on surgery day. Keep the faith, we are doing our best to do the same.

Thanks for caring,

Mark

F*ck Cancer

Written May 9, 2012 9:21p.m.

That's right, I saw that on a T-shirt on a website called "Zazzle," and it will be the first thing I order as soon as we get the "all clear" sign from the doctor tomorrow.

The facts for tomorrow: We arrive at 9 a.m. at the Mary Catherine Bunting Building at Mercy and then report to Nuclear Medicine. There, they will inject a dye that will eventually help determine which lymph node to remove and test to see if the cancer has spread. I'm here to tell you it has not. It will be the first bright spot on our journey to freedom from what should never have been.

Surgery is set to begin a few hours later. Dr. Neil Friedman will perform the double mastectomy and then come out to tell us how it all went. A short time later, Dr. Bernard Chang will perform the first phase of the reconstruction and then update us on the progress. And then, as long as everything goes right, which it will, Debbie will be in the recovery room and on the road to a real recovery.

There you go—it's all covered in four sentences, one paragraph. Seems simple. So why, when you read between the lines, does it hurt so much? Is it because I know my wife has already been through enough? Is it because you never understand, as many times as its explained to you, or how many articles and books you read, why bad things happen to good people? It's more painful to watch those you love the most suffer than to suffer yourself.

It's just not fair. I could never have imagined in my wildest dreams that seeing my wife take a shower tonight would be one of the saddest moments of my life. The same thing she does every day (and y'all should be so lucky to see it) was the last time I knew I would witness her like that ever again... and it broke my heart. Not because she will look any different in the end, not because she won't still be so incredibly beautiful, but because SHE has to go through the pain and suffering to be free of all of this.

My Debbie is a giver. But what she has gotten back the past few years, between losing her dad suddenly to cancer and now this, is not what is supposed to happen when you are always giving of yourself.

But all of this is out of our control, for any of us. The gift Debbie gets back tomorrow is the love of so many family and friends who will pack that waiting room. It's because she is constantly doing for others that they drop everything to be there for her. She deserves it. People love her. And those things ARE in our control. You can't think back on what has happened and why, you can't predict the future, but you can control how you live your life. My wife lives it to the fullest, because she cares. And that care has been returned in spades.

Thanks to so many who have already—and constantly—sent good wishes, prayers, and so, so much more. It has been overwhelming to witness, yet, at least from my perspective, because of the person she is, seems so fitting at the same time because Debbie does the same for others, when they are also facing misfortune and fear. I have never seen her back away from a challenge, or turn her back on a friend.

I have also learned, much more deeply than I ever realized, how women are truly affected by breast cancer. The mere mention of the words cements the bond that already exists between female friends and family and creates an instant connection to the stranger who might find out. They can immediately empathize, and everyone has a story. We are not the first to go through this, won't be the last. But the stories that are being written, page by page every day, are the ones of survival. And that is so friggin' cool. Together, everyone is making a difference.

Shock, surgery, survivor, the journey. Last week, after our doctor appointments, as we were waiting for the elevator, Debbie looked at me and told me she was "sorry" for putting me through this. That's a good one. The one that makes you pause, take a breath, collect yourself, and then come up with the answer that falls way short, "You must be kidding me, right? That's the silliest thing I've ever heard," I said. Whether she ever reads this or not, let me just say, that response didn't do her justice.

My real answer, if I could have come up with the right words, if I could get through it without breaking down, is to tell her this: "Deb, no matter what, I wouldn't have missed this for the world. This is where I was always meant to be from the first day I met you. I need you way more than you could ever need me. You give my life its meaning, and you have enriched it more than I could have ever hoped. You gave me my greatest gifts, our two beautiful daughters, who I marvel at every day. You are my motivation, my inspiration, my hope, my world, and my very best friend. You are a fighter. A hero. And I love you with all of my heart. And, I will see you on the other side of the surgery, my survivor.

I love you,

Mark

2 A Hero Rises

"YOU ARE A perfectly healthy 40-year–old woman, except you have breast cancer." That was what the nurse said to Debbie as she took her vital signs and checked her out, before it was time to head to the operating room. My girl was scared, but strong. She was confident and steadfast in her decision to go ahead with a double mastectomy, and what she believed, and I supported, as her best chance to beat the beast and be cancer free. Still, sitting in the pre-op room was one of the hardest moments of my life. I had to be strong, as well, but in the confines of my heart, I was hurting, I was sad, I was scared.

They pushed Debbie out of the pre-op room, and she sat in the hall for a moment to kiss everyone goodbye before it was time for her to head to the OR. Our kiss was brief, and it's not what I remember most. No, the image that will stay in my mind for all time was standing there as they rolled Debbie's wheelchair down the hall and into the unknown. It was almost too much to take. I knew at that moment our life would change. Debbie would be healthy, I could feel it, but I could also feel the unbearable feeling of helplessness as I watched her being rolled away, alone, left to face the greatest sacrifice she had ever made. Once she disappeared into the operating room, so did I, out of pre-op and into the privacy of the men's room... to cry.

All Clear!!

Written May 10, 2012 1:25 p.m.

Dr. Friedman says lymph nodes are negative!!!! First phase is done. What great news.

Time to order the F*ck Cancer shirts.

Thanks for caring,

Mark

The Road Ahead

Written May 10, 2012 4:27 p.m.

A new beginning. Cancer free (though we won't know 100% until the final pathology report next week, but all initial tests show lymph nodes are negative).

From Dr. Chang—reconstruction went perfectly. It went fast, as well! She has great "skin pockets," which means she's a terrific candidate for perfect implants. He put in the expanders and 50cc of fluid to get the process started, with more to come over the following weeks and months to stretch the tissue and muscle and prepare for implants. As if Deb wasn't hot enough before...

I saw her a little while ago in the recovery room, and while in a good deal of pain, she looks good. She will stay in recovery until the nurses and doctors believe she is ready to go upstairs... and the room is ready. 14th floor, but we don't know what room yet.

Many, many thanks to everyone who has supported and comforted us while we played the waiting game to get to surgery day. Thanks to all who have offered help and prayers. It has all paid off. The road to full recovery will not be a breeze; but being cancer free was always the ultimate goal, and it appears we have arrived. Thanks to all the family, especially Sharon and Alisa, who have suffered right along with Deb, worrying with her and for her. As mom and sister, I understand the bond... and I know that her pain was theirs every step of the way. And thanks to the many, many friends (our extended family) who have lent a helping hand already and kept us in your prayers. Our good friend, Debbie Rosenbaum, has a sign that hangs in her family room, my favorite one of all time: "Friends are the family you meet along the way." Indeed. We can never thank you enough.

This is all a huge relief. I needed this out of her, because now WE are in control and not held hostage to cells that have no place in anyone's body.

Once we are up in a room, I will update again. Keep the good vibes coming.

Thanks for caring,

Mark

Guestbook Entries:

Deb, I just received the update that your lymph nodes are all clear. I hope the worst will be behind you very soon. I love you, Mark, and your beautiful girls. You are loved by many, and you deserve all the health and happiness in the world. Stay strong, sarcastic and feisty.

Xoxo, Jennifer Spath

Soooo happy to hear the great news! We all did a little cheer here in rehab department when we heard! WE LOVE U, DEB.

XOXO, Mindi Neubauer

Debbie,

Gina and I were so happy to hear the positive results from today's surgery!!

When I see your posts and pictures on Facebook, I marvel at the true love and connection you and Mark so clearly share. What a gift when soul mates find each other.

I just finished reading Mark's updates on this site, and I was overwhelmed by his love and devotion for you. After talking with Gina and seeing all of the posts on this site, this much is overwhelmingly clear—you are an amazing mother, an incredible wife, a wonderful and giving friend, and an inspirational person. With all the love your husband, daughters, family, and friends have for you, I have no doubt that you will be feeling better and cancer free in no time.

My family and I will continue to pray for you and your family, and we wish you a speedy recovery.

Stephen Millstein

This is the best news!!! We are so happy all has gone well. Hugs and kisses to the whole Brodinsky family. I do believe a cocktail is in order. Have a great Mother's Day with your girls!!!!

All our love,

Marty, Sharon, Savannah and Jake Bass

It's All Good

Written May 10, 2012 9:53 p.m.

In a room now since about 7 p.m., and all is as well as can be expected. Deb is resting. There has been pain and nausea, but nothing unexpected. The pain is being controlled, the nausea comes and goes, but as of 11 p.m., she is resting.

Machines pump meds, leg warmers circulate the blood and make lots of little noises, and the TV volume is on low—the slight murmur of a news show. It's all secondary to watching Deb sleep, in the glow of the TV and the lights from the city twinkling outside the window, right near the JFX and Mercy Hospital. Peace is a good thing.

Cancer free. Good to say the words—if even to myself—because it means for the first time in nearly a month, I can sleep without wondering what this will all be like. Will it be "all clear" or will we learn there are more bad cells? We now have an answer. And it's all good. So Good Night.

Thanks for caring,

Mark

A Good Night
Written May 11, 2012 7:04 a.m.

Night at hospital wasn't as bad as I thought, though Debbie's first visit to the bathroom last night was a scene she won't ever want to repeat. She nearly passed out trying to walk there and barely made it back to the bed ... the surgery has taken so much out of her. The nurses visited almost every hour, and though she had a lot of nausea, Deb never got sick, and trips to the bathroom are getting a bit quicker to accomplish. She is still in a good deal of pain, but they are working on getting the pain meds just right. If all gets better, the goal is to get home later today.

Thanks again for all the well wishes. I am requesting no visitors at the hospital, and I will monitor how and when she can accept visitors at home this weekend. Rest is her best friend, and I know everyone wants to see her and to help, but we need to take it slow. Chaos and constant visitors won't do her any good, so please be respectful. Its Mother's Day weekend, and I want nothing more than for it to end on an up note with Deb really starting to feel better.

Thanks for caring,

Mark

Staying Ahead of Pain and Updates

Written May 11, 2012 10:30 a.m.

Still at the hospital, working on getting the pain management just right, so hopefully we can head home later today. The doctors changed up meds, and Deb is feeling less nauseous.

While writing the update, our breast surgeon, Dr. Friedman, just stopped by. He says all is going as expected, pain, nausea, light-headedness, if it happens, is just part of the process of "getting through it and getting better." Each day will be better than the last. Probably doesn't need the ringing endorsement, but the guy is good—great bedside manner, great doctor. Thankful we chose him.

Looking forward to getting home sometime today. Deb is very tired. Thanks for the check-ins. I am updating as fast and as much as possible. Much prefer you to read these—over phone calls—not going to answer many phone calls and can only return so many texts. Especially once we're home, it will take a lot to stay ahead of the pain, so if we ignore you—it's not on purpose. But I can provide updates on Caringbridge via the iPhone, so I will stay on top of that as much as possible. Keep the positive messages coming, been reading them to Deb, and it definitely makes a difference. We can feel the love and support.

Thanks for caring,

Mark

3 Battle Royale

THE SACRIFICE HAD been made. Now we waited for the final results.

Not on pins and needles in anticipation, mind you, especially not Debbie, who was too preoccupied with the pain and the drains. Those f*cking drains. I will never forget them. I despise them. They became the Achilles heel in the early weeks of recovery. These big, bulbous, blood-filled, plastic hell holes which kept Debbie tethered to the reminder of the toughest surgery of her life and held her captive, unable to realize true freedom on the road to recovery. It was like driving down the highway on a bicycle, pulling a truckload of concrete blocks behind you. Do I make myself clear?

The road to recovery from breast cancer surgery is filled with moments of gratitude and of fear. Periods of uncertainty, pangs of remorse, pauses for honest reflection ... and then there's the pain. Physical pain which still echoes today, embodied in the small pink heart pillows Debbie still keeps in our bed, and still slips beneath her armpit and the side of her breast when she goes to sleep. I'm not sure if the pangs of pain are real, or simply imagined, or if it's just a way to hold on to the thought of what once was. As in death, giving up a piece of yourself which is forever gone, you never get over it; you just get on with it.

There was much to learn about this time and no guide book, outside of the medical journals, to do it. Like raising children, there is no manual to deal with the emotional and physical consequences of this "overnight" surgery. Incredible how a few hours in time can change your world, for all time.

The crazy, amazing, and life-changing realization is we got good news ... but the words we so wanted to hear were just that—words. There was still so much, so much to overcome.

Dancing with the Devil
Written May 11, 2012 10:27 p.m.

Nice to be home. Deb is sleeping. Took another pain pill about an hour ago, then off to sleep. The hope is that she can make it through the night, peacefully. The hope is that every day gets a little bit better. The hope is the drain of "the drains" gets a little bit easier. I noticed tonight when it was time for the procedure to empty those drains how Deb closed her eyes for a time. Though I couldn't see, I knew behind those closed eyes was sadness for having had to give up a part of herself to the beast. It's never easy to fight, even when you win. And make no mistake, we have won. But we have also sacrificed to do it. We believe she is now cancer free, but, man, this is far from over.

I believe cancer is like dancing with the Devil. In this case, the Devil went down... but not to Georgia. He's done. But there are more battles out there, battles yet to be fought and won, fought and lost. Cancer seems to force sacrifice, whether you win or lose. You give up part, or all, of yourself. Few are left unscarred, yet underneath, you also get something back. A part of you that you might not have known existed, a part of you that reached back for something extra, that refused to give in, that stood its ground, and win or lose, you battled like a champ.

Deb's a champ, a winner, and the future is now so bright. But you will always look back and remember.

You'll remember a time before you were told it was time to fight, a time when you were scared and helpless, a time when all you wanted to do was turn and run, rather than face the tough choice, a time when doctor visits, tests, biopsies, pathology, surgery, and recovery were something that "other people" dealt with. Until it was your turn.

So you remember, but you also look forward. You grasp hold of the new attitude and outlook you have on life, and you run with it, not away from it. You never forget, but now you have earned the right to make new memories. You get to live another day, many, many more days, with pride. I'm so proud of Debbie. She made the sacrifice. She showed the courage. She, for the sake of her family, gave up to get.

So F*ck Cancer. F*ck the Devil. Celebrate Life. And we will. Get ready.

Thanks for caring,

Mark

Guestbook Entries:

Debbie, You are a warrior, a survivor, and profoundly brave. You have people praying for you all over the country that you've never met, but who care about you, anyway. And I can't wait to tell you in person how much I admire your strength.

Mark, thank you for your candid, heartfelt posts in the journal. They help us to know how she's doing, but also touch our hearts with the love & admiration you have for Debbie. I feel blessed just from having read your messages of love & hope.

Please let us know if there's anything we can do to help in the days & weeks ahead.

Jen Margerum

I just found out about this site today. I had no doubt you would get great news after the surgery. Keeping the Brodinsky family in my thoughts and prayers. Deb, you are one tough cookie, and I hope your recovery continues to be smooth and uneventful. Mark, your words are beautiful and your love for Debbie is amazing. I know you are all supported by a fantastic network of family and friends, but if you need anything, please know we are willing and able to help! XOXO Lisa and Erik

Lisa Sparks

Sleeping Through

Written May 12, 2012 9:53 a.m.

Deb had a pretty good night. She slept from 10 p.m. to 8 a.m., with only a wake-up at 5 a.m. for a pain pill. No pain, no gain. Part of the healing process. She did her exercises for the day and took her first shower since surgery. All of it takes a lot out of her, though, so it's time again for rest.

Thanks for caring,

Mark

Mother's Day / Full Circle

Written May 13, 2012 7:20 a.m.

Late update: Having fun at the Gorman's Bat Mitzvah will do that to you. Had to sleep in just a bit. Gorman family, thanks for throwing such a fantastic party to honor your beautiful Asia. We had a blast; it was wonderful and truly felt like a celebration of so many things. It gave us a chance to blow off some of the stress of the past month. And thank you even more for including Debbie's video message to Asia. She would have given the world to be there, but the bottom line is now she will be there for all the good times to come!!

Deb had what I would consider a good day yesterday. Thanks to everyone who is paying attention and allowing her to get her rest. She slept a lot yesterday, all good. She is still in some pain. We'd be surprised if she wasn't, but it is being pretty well controlled by the medications, and she is improving. She slept through the night last night and didn't ask for a pain pill until 6 a.m. Seven hours of peace.

From her first steps after surgery to try and get to the bathroom, when she was shaking uncontrollably, to last night, when I was sent a picture of her SITTING on the sofa eating sushi, we are making great progress. Thanks to Cindy and Jeff Schreiber for staying with her last night while the rest of the family attended the Bat Mitzvah. You can't imagine how comforting it was to us to know she was in such caring and "professional" hands. Thank you, Dr. Schreiber, for handling the drain change last night. Thanks to Deb, who insisted the girls and I attend the Bat Mitzvah, no matter what.

So, May 13th, 2012, Mother's Day, 2012—truly a celebration for Deb, for all of us. It was April 13th when we got the news the biopsy was "not benign," and today, her first Mother's Day post surgery, she is cancer free.

We have come full circle. Words can never do justice for the joy we are experiencing, family and our extended family (our friends), knowing that this Mother's Day, Debbie is healthy. Cancer free. No more cloud of worry about suspicious mammograms (nothing to be concerned about), MRI's that show something "unusual" (but everything's fine, right?), ultrasounds that "don't show a thing," and finally biopsies ("from looking at the tissue sample, it's a 1-in-10 chance it's malignant," we were told). This part is all behind us.

What's in front of us is hope and joy. There is work to be done. Easy for me to say, because I'm not the patient, but I will be there every step of the way, making sure the healing goes as planned, that the pain subsides, that the reconstruction is just what Deb wants it to be. She deserves the best. She is strong, resilient. I am in awe of her ability to handle all of this with grace and courage.

Debbie, from the bottom of our hearts, Sophie, Emily, and I just want to say thanks. Thanks for being the person we knew you are and even more than the person we know you are. You have shown us, and everyone, what it means to be brave, what it means to have hope and resolve. You have taken it all in stride, made the tough decision and never, ever looked back. Even today, only a few days into your recovery, your ability to handle the pain and the "procedures," barely shedding a tear and showing incredible strength, is a tribute to the incredible person you are. Your dedication, devotion, and love for our family have stood a tremendous test, and you aced it, with flying colors.

Happy Mother's Day. Can't wait to spend today, and all the days of my life, with you. My hero. My survivor. I love you.

Thanks for caring,

Mark

No Pain? Real Gain
Written May 14, 2012 9:48 a.m.

9 a.m. Monday: Debbie slept through the night. Fell asleep about 9:30 before it was time for her next pain pill at 11 p.m.

and woke up about 7 a.m. Then fell back asleep about 7:30 and still sleeping. So we are going on 16 hours without asking for pain medicine. Incredible. Only 3-1/2 days removed from surgery. When we emptied the drains at 7 a.m., one side was already starting to look a lighter shade. All good.

We have some goals for the week ahead. We hope things continue to improve and the drains can be removed by the end of the week. That's the first HUGE step in the right direction for more physical freedom. It's a big weekend. Sophie's dance recital is Saturday night, and I know Deb really wants to go. Then Sunday evening, we have tickets to Lady Antebellum and Darius Rucker at Merriweather Post. I bought those tickets for her back on Valentine's Day, never imagining what might lie ahead. For her to be able to attend both events would be awesome. Lady A is one of our favorite groups. Doc said 7-10 days on drain removal normally. If it's 10 days, she would still have those in for this weekend. We'll see.

Let's think positive, drain free by Friday.

Was a really good Mother's Day for Deb. Family came over for about 3 hours for dinner, provided by the Wachs family. Thanks to all of them, and especially Melissa, who asked me just the night before at the Gorman Bat Mitzvah about bringing food for Sunday night. She insisted, and it was delicious. Debbie was happy to be with the family, and it obviously wore her out. Sleep is a good thing. Healing is even better.

Sophie, Emily, and I gave Deb a "pink ribbon" necklace for Mother's Day. Thanks to Marley and Todd Brown at Radcliffe for helping me design it.

And, as always, thanks for caring.

Mark

Bump in the Road

Written May 14, 2012 10:31 p.m.

No one ever said it would be easy. As positive as the day/night was on Mother's Day, the day after was different. It started out well, with no pain meds needed until about 9 a.m.... but then things changed.

Debbie's mom was over for the day to help out, and I elected not to go into the office (maybe tomorrow); it ended up being the right move. A late morning shower turned into an adventure. I was downstairs while Sharon assisted Debbie just outside the shower upstairs. Next thing I know, I hear my name being called, loudly, in a panic. I rush up to see Debbie slumped down in the shower, the water still beating down on her, and her mom holding onto Deb with one hand to keep her from hitting the shower floor. Debbie passed out. It probably lasted for less than 15 seconds, but seemed like an eternity. She finally came around as we pulled her out and got her dried off. Doc explained it as a consequence to major surgery—says you can't get out of bed too quick, you need to drink more and more liquids, a warm shower lowers your BP, anyway, and the pain meds don't do you any favors.

There's that medical explanation again; it all seems so logical afterward. But when your wife, who gave up both her breasts just four days ago, is slumped over in the bottom of your shower... logic isn't the first thing that crosses your mind. First you act, then you react, and then you relive it all during story time.

A few hours later, there was a huge blood stain along the side of what I call Deb's breast vest... we thought one of the drain "bulbs" was leaking, only to learn after cleaning her up that she was leaking. Blood was running down from the place where the drain tube enters her body. Doc says it can happen, some blood clots form and then open... and the blood can drip out right next to the cord and down the side. There's that logic again. Good to know each event can be explained. Makes me feel much better... I should just carry around a post-mastectomy medical book, so I can read right along as the "previously unexplained" events play out. Hope it includes pictures!

The 2 to 3 times a day "changing" of the drains is interesting enough. For anyone who has experienced it, you learn what true love is. Then again, I was there when my bride gave birth to two daughters, so let's put everything in perspective. You know the biggest difference, though? At one event, she was giving up blood to give life... this time the blood she gives is from saving her own. Kind of gives you chills.

The day got under control after that. More liquids, move slower, eat more, wean off the powerful pain meds if she can handle it. Why not, she's handled everything else with grace and dignity. Not sure one day who will show a crack in the armor first, her or me. Probably me. I know I've said it before, watching those you love hurt might be worse than hurting yourself. Next to watching Debbie's dad pass away right before my eyes in a hospital room 2-1/2 years ago, seeing her slumped over in the shower, four days removed from breast surgery, ranks right up there on the scale of things I will never, ever forget.

It's all part of the journey. I recently looked up the word journey, "the act of traveling from one place to another, a trip." Those last two words seem to sum it up well. It's a trip alright, though I have no doubt the final destination will be worth the work it took to get there. The most satisfying moments in life are the ones you struggle to achieve. If you've never been down, you can never experience the joy of getting back up. We'll be back up soon enough.

Thanks for caring,

Mark

A Better Day

Written May 16, 2012 5:17 a.m.

A better day for Debbie on Tuesday. Thanks to our friends, Lisa and Jill, who stayed with Deb for most of the day, while I went back to work for a few hours. Deb was alert and had no major incidents, except for feeling a little light-headed at one point, which she noticed and took precautions to lie down before anything happened. The pain is still manageable, and she was on regular Tylenol and Motrin during the day before asking for the "stronger" stuff at night, following another shower.

Fearful of another shower fainting incident, this time, I helped. We used a shower stool, and I got in with her. I'm starting to get a better feel for what it would be like to care for someone in a long-term care situation. This won't be long-term, but the circumstances and the round-the-clock care are darn close. Not complaining by any means, just noticing the similarities.

The drains seem to be improving; we are monitoring the amount of blood flowing into them and the color of that blood. (It's all a long story.) There is a doctor's appointment tomorrow (Thursday) afternoon. If the drain situation continues to improve, they are removed. If not, they stay at least into next week. Let's hope for the best. Getting rid of those dreaded drains will mean mobility and freedom. We'll see. Deb will at least get to lose the medicine ball and pouch she has had to carry around like a ball and chain for the past week. Though she may miss the pain medicine that gets pumped from the ball!!

All in all, not a bad day. The goal is more strength and mobility by the weekend to attend a few events ... Sophie's dance recital and the Lady Antebellum concert on Sunday, both which I checked and have confirmed handicap seating if necessary to make things a bit more comfortable. We'll see. First, Debbie needs the energy to attend those events. We can't sacrifice good health to get there.

Here's to good health!! Thanks for caring,

Mark

Cancer Free!

Written May 16, 2012 9:47 a.m.

CANCER FREE. I think, next to "it's a boy" or "it's a girl," they may be the two words I most wanted to hear in my life. We just got the call from Dr. Friedman, all pathology reports are in and it's official, all clear!!

The right breast had ductal cancer and a tumor about 3mm—the left breast is benign. There were two sentinel lymph nodes and one other lymph node removed—and all are clear! Dr. Friedman believes because Deb chose a double mastectomy, there may be no other treatment necessary, not even Tamoxifen. We will meet with a medical oncologist after our meeting with Dr. Friedman on June 13th. He said no rush.

What great news. What a relief. Pretty f*cking excited, if you know what I mean. I answered the phone when Friedman called, but I could tell he didn't want to tell me, he wanted to tell the patient himself. I had to wake Debbie up for the call. :) Debbie deserved to hear the good news firsthand. The highest peak in the journey so far. Emotions are high. Need time to reflect later, right now just reason to celebrate. It's 5 o'clock somewhere!!!!

Thanks for caring,

Mark

Guestbook Entries:

Dearest Debbie & Mark,

Am at work and first chance I have had to sign the guestbook since I texted you this morning. Still am choked up and prayers have been answered! This is the first sigh of relief in weeks. Whatever word more than ECSTATIC would be, that is what we want to say. Will call you around noontime today. We love you so, so, so very much always!

Bonnie & Robin Brodinsky (Mom & Dad)

FABULOUS, THE VERY BEST NEWS & IT MADE MY DAY!!!!!

Marilyn Lefkowitz

What a terrific phone call you received this morning!! Fantastic news!!! What joyous words!!! We are so ecstatic for you, Debbie!! Just wonderful!!!!!!! We love you!!!!!

Margi Granek

Reflect & Move Forward

Written May 16, 2012 9:12 p.m.

After the unbelievably great news this morning, I kept hoping my F*ck Cancer T-shirt would show up in the mail... no such luck. Maybe tomorrow.

Such a great day for news, and mostly a good day for recovery. Deb was up way too much today, didn't get enough zzzz's in and paid the price tonight—she's exhausted and needed a pain pill, after a day of only Tylenol and Motrin. We were hoping tomorrow's doctor visit with Dr. Chang's PA (Physician's Assistant) would be the day we get the drains removed, but the signs are not positive for that change.

The "fluid" levels have not been consistently at or below where they should be (meaning less drainage), and the color is not light enough, either. Unless there's a miracle in the morning, I don't hold out much hope the drains will come out tomorrow. What sucks is if not tomorrow, then not until Monday at the earliest, because the office is not available on Friday. That means a weekend with those plastic bubbles still hanging around. Again, no one said this would be perfect. But after this morning's news, it's hard to be negative.

Then again, I'm not the one with tubes coming out of my body on both sides, and I'm not the one in pain... at least physically. Emotionally, well, let's just say I'm thankful for the journal. And I apologize for the sometimes extended entries, but it gives me a place to write down my thoughts and air out my emotions—a place to reflect at night, or relive the prior day in the morning. Without it, I'm not sure how the stress and experiences of the past month would have affected me.

I believe, for Debbie, the relief of post-surgery and this morning's news (she was in tears as soon as she hung up the phone with the doctor... such relief) have obviously meant so much. But tonight there was the first hint of how this is all getting old quickly. Deb wants the drains out, wants to feel like a real person, is getting a bit weary of the whole process. She's tired of being tired. Who can blame her?

But, Debbie, I can tell you one thing for sure: this morning's phone call was vindication of the toughest decision of your life. It was always your call, and you made the right one. How many people take that chance in life and get it right? You're awesome for your determination and your bravery. So many people love and respect you for how you have handled yourself during this very difficult time, and it only reinforces how they feel about you. Just look at the outpouring of love—cards, gifts, meals, and a ton of attention. We can never thank everyone enough for stepping up and stepping forward to help. It is overwhelming and touching beyond belief.

So part of the journey is over. Still a long way to go, but we have a lot more control than we did at this time last week, on the eve of the surgery. Debbie made the sacrifice to beat cancer, and it paid off. What I've learned is you ALWAYS sacrifice something when it comes to the "C" word. Either you go through chemotherapy, radiation, lose a body part, or worse, you're done. No matter what, you will give up some part of yourself, some part of your freedom, some part of what was your good health, and go through hell to defeat the f*cker. Some win, some lose. Your attitude, your determination, and then some help from the man upstairs all combine to draw up the outcome. If you want to use the word miracle... I'm good.

So tomorrow we take the show back on the road, back to the Breast Center at Mercy for a follow-up. Strength, determination, hope, fear, all come back into play. Except now we're in control. We and the doctors make the calls now. Cancer has no place here. The only "C" word I need to type now as I say good night is thanks for "c"aring.

Mark

Last Dance

Written May 17, 2012 9:48 p.m.

So, Donna Summer proves my point. Sometimes you win, sometimes you lose. Cancer forces sacrifice; the Queen of Disco paid with her life. Cancer got the best of her. Not so here.

Today was a follow-up visit with Dr. Chang's PA, Meg. Very nice woman, but it pretty much went the way we expected.

The medicine ball, which was now empty, anyway, is gone. The drains are still draining, so they stay. Looking at the levels, neither Deb nor I thought they would be coming out. It's okay, they need to do their work; you can't remove them too early and then have your body fill up with blood/fluid.

Yes, it's only been a week. Yes, there needs to be patience. Yes, we've heard the stories about 10 to 14 days or more before the drains can be pulled out. Yes, we know it's for the best. Medicine, science, doctor's orders, logical steps, it all makes perfect sense. But isn't it okay for Debbie to still feel sad and disappointed?

We were driving home from the doctor appointment today, right around the same time her surgery was beginning last week. For the first time since she was ready to head back to the OR, I witnessed her crying. On the drive home today, as she explained to our good friend, Marni, about today's appointment, she broke into tears. She knew going in there was little doubt nothing would change today, she remembers the great news we got yesterday morning about the cancer being gone, she knows she has so much to be thankful for. But she was still disappointed today. She's allowed to feel sad—heck, she's allowed to feel so much more. Only the 2nd time she's really shed tears in a week?? My girl is strong, let her emote, let her experience frustration and be impatient. Let her need to have a good cry. It's okay. There's nothing to be ashamed of. It's not easy. We/she knows the best is ahead, she feels the love and support from everyone, she knows the end of the journey will be worth it. Still, it's okay to give in to the moment once in a while; it's ok to be human. It's okay to NOT be okay once in a while. It's okay, Deb.

Debbie is up and awake a lot more. Each day does get just a bit better, even with some mild setbacks. We're looking forward to a nice weekend. Emily pitches multiple innings tomorrow at her softball game, and Debbie hopes to witness a few of them. Saturday night, Sophie has her dance recital, and this year it is close by, so Deb hopes to go and see her dance. Sunday night, Debbie and I have tickets to see Darius Rucker and Lady Antebellum at Merriweather Post. If she rests up all day, I believe she can do it. I know she really wants to go. That's our goal.

I remember texting Debbie a few weeks back (April 21st), telling her I just saw the Lady "A" video on TV and their concert will be one of our first milestones after surgery. She texted me back "it's a deal." I still have the text. I'm ready if she is.

Let the weekend begin. Hope the T-shirt shows up. Hope my beautiful bride keeps feeling better and better. Hope the plastic drain bubbles get lighter and lighter. Hope we make it to everything Deb wants to do. Hope everyone has a terrific weekend. Hope Donna Summer will RIP.

Thanks for caring, Mark

Weekend Wrap

Written May 20, 2012 11:03 p.m.

As Meatloaf sings: "2 out of 3 ain't bad"....

Deb made it to 2 of the 3 goals she set for the weekend: Sophie's dance recital on Saturday and the Lady Antebellum/ Darius Rucker/Thompson Square concert we saw Sunday night. The only thing she missed was Emily playing softball, but there will be more games to come (though Emily did pitch the final inning Saturday afternoon—and made a throw to home plate that ended the game with the bases loaded! I was so sorry Deb missed that one.) Sophie's recital and the Lady A concert were one or done events. Btw—Sophie and her friends were phenomenal dancers in their performance at the JCC Gordon Center. Kudos to the girls.

So progress has been made. Debbie managed to get out for both events. Saturday night, it was only for about 90 minutes, and it was taxing for her. For Sunday's concert, she had to sleep/rest all day just to make the attempt, and we still left the show with a few songs to go—but Lady A was the final act and we left at 10:15 p.m.—Deb had had enough. I am so proud of her for making the effort—I know in my heart she did it as much for me as for herself (maybe more for me, since she knew I bought the tickets for Valentine's Day). Debbie was a real trooper. She still had to pop some Motrin and a pain pill during the shows... just to get through. But she did it, and we accomplished what we promised each other we would try to do before her surgery, which was to make it to that concert.

Her drain levels are slowly going down, and right now we are right at the mark we need to be (better to actually be below the mark), but we need 48 hours of good readings to get the go-ahead to have the doctors remove the drains. Patience. That's something we are learning together.

I will say that with a weekend full of events, I have gained a new appreciation for the things that matter most. It might sound cliché to say when you get a scare, you start to pay attention to everything that matters—but so what—if that's what happens, if the little moments become the big focus and they linger longer in your mind, so what. It pays to pay attention to the things that really matter—and to make a mental note not to forget the things that should be unforgettable. But the things that happen in the blink of an eye are sometimes, unfortunately, forgotten just as quickly.

The week ahead will be more rest and the little exercises to keep Debbie from getting stiff, as well as some short walks to keep everything loose and gain back some stamina. We'll see how the drain situation goes.

We did have a moment on Saturday night—one of those times that all we could do was look at each other and be silent. In between dance performances, waiting for Sophie's group to come on, Debbie was shuffling through pictures on her phone, only to come across the one we had taken shortly after her biopsy. The doctors had done a number on her right breast when they took the tissue sample, and it created a hematoma. That was why we took the picture. But when she saw it and showed it to me, I could only look at it and then at her—and say nothing—just give her a half-smile. What's there to say, the past is the past now—it hurts, but there are plenty of things you are forced to look back on in life and feel the sense of sadness, even for a moment. Yet life is full of renewal, so when you feel the twinge of pain from the past, you focus on what you have to be fortunate for right now, hold it close, and look toward tomorrow and a brighter future. It gets to feel brighter, too, because you made it through the tough time and now have an appreciation for life on the other side. It's all going to be fine—I'm glad I'm along for the ride. I wouldn't want it any other way.

For me, this is where I was always meant to be, where I am needed, and it feels good to be needed—for whatever might come our way.

Thanks for your strength and determination this weekend, Deb. These ARE the moments you don't forget.

I love you, Debbie.

Thanks for caring,

Mark

Guestbook Entries:

My thoughts and prayers are hugging Debbie and you, Mark.

I just learned about your journey when I logged into Facebook today, and then read all of your journal entries. Your words are so honest and true. Your passion and love for Debbie and sharing the details of this challenge show an amazing courage on your part. No wonder both are you are such good partners: you face life head-on together.

I know you have a lot of family and friends who are there for you, but please count me among them if you need ANYTHING!! Love to both of you,

Helene King

Dear Deb and Mark,

We were so happy to read that the recital and concert were events that you both were able to attend, and, Mark, how prolific your writings are, perhaps a new career is on the horizon. It is so heartwarming to read about the journey you and Deb have been going through together—it is never easy to deal with such a difficult situation, but thank God, the future is clear and full of sunny days ahead-we hope those drains do come out soon and that Deb will be more comfortable. Thanks for the update!

Hugs, Reva and Bernard Suffel

So sorry that this next lap in the journey is not going as quickly as we would all want for you, but it is so moving to read about how you each take such good care of each other. Mark, your care giving is much more active, but Deb's strength and determination is in part a way of taking care of you and your precious union. I am in awe.

Gail Kass

Deb, I think about you all the time, hoping every day gets better & better.

Mark, thanks so much for all the updates and being the wonderful person that you are!!

Debe Moore

(D)rain, (D)rain, Go Away

Written May 21, 2012 10:23 p.m.

Seems like it's been coming down forever. Outside the rain has stopped for now... but inside the drains, well, they keep pouring. It seems like I focus on it a lot, but it has become the Achilles heel of the recovery, because they represent the true remnants of the surgery. We are 10 days out of the hospital now, but it's like an umbilical cord that keeps you attached to that place. It's the one thing I know Debbie hates and the one thing I know that once they are removed, she will feel like she is in the next stage of her recovery. However, we are not there yet. The drain levels are maintaining, not waning.

How come I know it's a big deal? I know because when I went to empty them tonight, she put her head on my shoulder and started to cry. The place where they enter her body is sore. Add to that the daily pain of the breast expanders, which press on her ribs, stretch her chest muscles, and sometimes make her feel like she can't breathe... and well, you get the picture. So what do you do? You rest and try to remain distracted. When you are lying around in pain, it ain't easy.

I don't mean to say things are awful—they are not. We had dinner as a family tonight! Many thanks to Judy, Gary, Laura, Danny, Tracey, and Jason for the delicious meal. I didn't make a big deal to the girls about Debbie joining us at the table, but it didn't take long for Sophie to bring it up—and you could tell they both loved to see their mom sitting across from them at dinner. Besides the good meal, Deb had a good day, she was awake a bit too much—that's right, I'm paying attention—but all in all, it was a good day.

Each day goes by much more quickly now than it did when all we did was try to stay busy and NOT think about the cancer or the pending surgery. But the days now are filled with work—doing everything a "single" parent would have to do. Respect to all those who live that life every day... caring for kids, working a job (my business), and keeping the house in order. But here's the rub—add to all of that the job of caring for someone who can't do much for themselves and you add a layer of responsibility that, to me, changes the whole dynamic. But—and I'm serious about this—I'm not complaining; I'm just explaining. It is a labor of love; if I can't step up and be there for Debbie and my family in a time of need, then I don't deserve the same love and respect in return. I am learning what it's like to handle what I refer to as a "short-term" care case. I am gaining the utmost respect for those who care for their loved ones in long-term care AND still try to run a family.

I do have a complaint, however. Everyone has been great, sending food, food credits, flowers, gifts, and the gift of their time and attention to Debbie (more on that some other time). But what I'm worried about are the desserts. Cookies, cakes, muffins, chocolates, blendies, Italian ice, mandel bread, etc. My fear is that there won't be just one pair of breasts coming along soon, there will be two—Debbie's new ones AND my man boobs!! We gotta get this stuff out of the house. Cancer will be an afterthought once the diabetes from all this sugar kicks in. Wow.

Anyway, I'm tired, like most nights. Whose decision was it to do these updates before bed, anyway? I've got another full day ahead!! Here's to another day of healing. F*ck the drains ;)

Thanks for caring,

Mark

Game On!

Written May 22, 2012 11:21 p.m.

A major milestone tonight as Debbie was able to attend Emily's softball game in Lutherville. It was a big win against the first place team in our age group, 9-10 girls. So glad Deb got to see the victory. I co-manage, and it was one of our best games of the season. Deb even got to see Emily pitch the final inning. By the time the game was over, though, Deb was more than ready to get home and get to sleep. The outing made her tired, but at least she got to go. So there were two victories on the night!!!

Overall, it was a good day for Deb. We got a call from the plastic surgeon's office asking us to come in on Thursday morning. They want to do a check, especially with the long holiday weekend coming up, and there is the possibility, I stress possibility, that the drains will be removed. We're hopeful. Like I haven't mentioned it before, but Debbie is waaaaaaaaaay over the drains and the whole cleaning process. She's worried also that the longer the drains remain in her body, the increased risk for infection. I'm sure, however, the doctors also are aware—and all will be discussed on Thursday.

Thanks to the friends who came to help and visit today, and thanks to Marni for taking Deb out for a pedicure. I know it made her feel better.

BTW, more cookies arrived today. Help me, somebody please help me.

Thanks for caring,

Mark

The More Things Stay the Same
Written May 24, 2012 11:04 a.m.

No change. No go. Doctor (or doctor's PA to be exact) says the drains stay, at least until Tuesday (because of the Memorial Day weekend), and will ONLY be removed then if levels are where they should be. However, next Thursday is D-Day—now called Drain Day around here, no matter what.

Debbie is disappointed, but it's far from unexpected. We are getting close to where the drain levels should be—but we're not there yet. I was a bit more hopeful the doctors would see we were a bit close with one of them and remove it, but it didn't happen. I know the drains are making Deb sore, but she's not a sore loser—she figured it would go like this today, anyway.

So at least 5-7 days more of the same routine. Woulda been nice to see them come out and have a little freedom—on the same weekend we honor those brave men and women who have given their lives to protect our own. But it's not to be.

"It's only a few more days." If you know Debbie—a word of warning—do yourself a favor and don't say those words to her, since you're not the person walking around with them hanging out of your body. She's tired and sick of them, though she had a very positive attitude when we got the news this morning. She knew before the PA even walked in the room—because Deb heard her talking in the hallway—asking for assistance to remove the drains, only to say "never mind" as she looked at the daily tracking chart we had turned in.

It's been two weeks since this all went down. I told her this morning it's hard to believe it has been that long—time has flown by—and at the same time, it has crept along—if that makes any sense. Debbie responded to me, "It feels more like two years." Believe me, I get it.

It has certainly been two weeks filled with more stress (surgery day and the first day home), joy (pathology - cancer free), sadness (sense of loss, the drains), and love (us, the girls, family, friends) than I could have ever imagined you could pack into a 14-day period. I wouldn't trade a single second, because it is what life is all about.

Debbie is getting through. But getting through because of a solid foundation of family, friends, support, and herself—my love—who is just one of the greatest patients you have ever seen. She rarely feels sorry for herself, she doesn't cry often, she still has a sense of humor, she takes the pain, the discomfort, the worry, and the day-to-day healing all in stride. Deb has made this first part of the journey what it is—tolerable ... and then some. I can't thank her enough for being the person she is. She makes me proud to be her husband. She made the sacrifice, she got up off the mat to battle the recovery period, and she is handling the challenge of getting out and getting on with life. She does it all with grace, strength, perseverance, and a great attitude for life. And to top it all off, she's still smokin' hot. :) You can't give me a better package than that—I'm a lucky guy.

I love you, Deb. Never change. The best is yet to come.

Thanks for caring,

Mark

Feeling Better and Giving Thanks

Written May 25, 2012 9:27 p.m.

Not a bad day for Debbie. Plenty of friends and food this Friday. Not much time to rest, though, so by the end of the Oriole's game tonight, Deb had had enough. A good win will do that to you. :)

The big news tonight—Deb pretty much showered herself—not easy when you are standing there holding drains in one hand and soap in another. But she even managed to wash her hair! Not bad for a girl who a little more than a week ago was slumped over in the shower. So proud of Debbie. She is the one taking the initiative to do some more things for herself. I'm not surprised, though—that's how she rolls.

That's the update, but on the eve of a weekend to reflect and remember those who protect our freedom, I also wanted to take a moment to give thanks to some of those who have helped Debbie and my family so much over the past two weeks:

Lisa and Jill, who have been at our home almost every day for more than a week to help with some basic chores, laundry, dishes, organization, keeping Deb company, and allowing me to get out and go to work, cause if I don't, we don't eat. 100% commission sales will do that to you. :)

To Marni, who took Debbie for her first pedicure, post-surgery (her first time out of the house), then "took on" the very personal task of helping to shower Debbie a few times the past few weeks. If that's not love, friend to friend, I don't know what is.

To Jenny, who keeps Debbie laughing every day and made us a delicious pre-surgery dinner. She tells the best stories, and there's always drama going on in her life, so the stories keep coming.

To Deb's sister, Alisa, who has been there every step of the way. I know it's not easy for her, living more than 40 minutes away from her little sister in need. She can't always be here in person, but she is always checking in to make sure things are going okay. She even made time in the middle of her busy day to take Sophie to her 12-year-old check-up, and then picked up a trunk full of "stuff" we needed—including wine and beer!! She used to be referred to as Mother Superior, because of the way she looked out for and worried about Debbie too much when they were younger, but in these past few weeks, Alisa has been just that—"superior"—not just in her love and devotion to Debbie, but for the way she has held herself together throughout the entire ordeal. As Alisa reminded us today, Debbie has pretty much been in some kind of pain since the agonizing biopsy on April 11th. I know it has pained Alisa as much to watch her sister go through this—almost as much as Mom.

Which brings me to Sharon—Mom. What can I say? They say you don't know what someone is really about until you walk a mile in their shoes. Sharon has been here before, a 20-year breast cancer survivor herself. It has been too difficult for me to put myself in her place and think how she must feel watching her baby girl go through all of this. All I know is Sharon is strong and courageous in her own right—as I've talked about before, Debbie is the same, proof the apple doesn't fall far from the tree. Thanks, Mom, for everything, and sometimes, for just being there.

Oh yeah, and what about those two other girls in my life, Sophie and Emily? Our daughters have been just great. I know they were scared and fearful at first when their mom told them she had cancer. But we reassured them she wasn't going anywhere and the surgery would make her better in the long run. I have to say my girls have really been so well behaved and supportive. It has made everything easier. Maybe we are actually doing something right.

Me? I'm just along for the ride. I'm trying to do what anyone would—step up—and do what it takes to keep everything and everyone moving forward, and caring for my love as I know she would do for me. No questions asked, no complaints. But I could not have done it all without help—just some of which I mentioned above. It's been a long two months—coming off vacation in early April, immediately followed by the biopsy, the diagnosis, waiting for surgery, the double mastectomy, post-surgery, recovery... it's been one hell of a rollercoaster ride.

It's far from over, and I could never, ever mention everyone who has contributed to this recovery. I'm not trying to leave anyone out... you have all made a HUGE difference. Every friend, family member (even acquaintances) who have sent messages of love and support, sent food (oy the sweets), food credits, flowers, clothing, donations, we thank you all so much. It becomes difficult to put into words what I really want to say to everyone. We are truly blessed.

This is a weekend where plenty of families and friends (the family we meet along the way) will be together to enjoy the holiday. Time to relax, and reflect on those who have made the ultimate sacrifice, to keep us safe. Thanks to the veterans, the fallen heroes—and in these past few weeks, right in our own home, thanks to the heroes who kept my wife not only sane, but safe and sound. We will never forget. Thanks for caring,

Mark

Goal and Good Night

Written May 26, 2012 10:00 p.m.

Hot day—the heat can take its toll on even the "healthiest" of people. Today, it wiped Deb out—after being outside for only an hour. It was worth it, though, because we got to see our big girl, Sophie, score a goal at her soccer game today. Debbie decided to make the trip out to Hampstead to see her play, but the game was at 1:30 in the afternoon, and even after sitting in the shade, she was wiped out ... came home and took a 2-1/2 hour nap.

We were also able to get out of the house again this evening, with dinner over at our neighbors and good friends, the Carswell's. It was delicious, as always. Deb was even able to cut her own flank steak—might not seem like an amazing feat, but using those arm and shoulder muscles, that's a big accomplishment. Right before we left for dinner, Deb was even able to lift her arms and put a ponytail in her hair. Whoever thought that simple act could cause pain... but she got it done. No surprise. Give her a goal, she'll get there.

After a couple of hours at the Carswell's home, I could tell Deb had had enough; she was tired. She offered me the opportunity to hang out there, while she went home to shower and get ready for bed. Of course, I agreed—NOT. Did she really think

I was letting her go home by herself, shower, and get ready for bed? Not on your life. I'm in this to win it.

I will say, more and more, Debbie's been talking about being "flat." For her, I'm sure it's a tough, emotional concept to grasp, especially when you look in the mirror and see nothing but scars and skin pockets. I honestly don't give it a second thought. I think she looks adorable, and it won't be long before things are "getting filled in and filled out," if you know what I mean.

Doesn't matter, though—flat breasts, medium, big... I love her just the same. I understand her uncertainty, and, believe me, I can appreciate the emotional journey she is on—not just physically, but mentally. I think though once the drains are out and more saline is in, she'll start to see how this will all come together. The pieces will start to fit, the pain will subside, the new body will take shape. I can only hope it is everything Deb wants and more, because she deserves it. She is making a bold drive down a scary road, but she is headed in the right direction. May all the lights on this road be green, may the road be mostly smooth, may the final destination be exactly where she wants to go. I'm the one riding shotgun now; Deb's in the driver's seat. The cancer is nothing but road kill.

Can't wait to put the pedal to the metal—and get well.

Thanks for caring,

Mark

Guestbook Entries:

Dear Debbie and Mark,

I read Mark's journal about your journey and am amazed at how magnificently he writes; this journal should truly be made into a book. It is a real love story that touches our hearts and souls each time we read. Have a peaceful weekend, and, yes, we ALL have so much to be grateful for, may all of the days, months, and years ahead bring each of you health and happiness in abundance. Please give Deb a big kiss from us. She is quite THE WOMAN!

Love, Reva and Bernard

I just read all of the entries & all I can say is "wow!" Deb, you are an amazing, strong, kind, and beautiful woman! I have always said that you are one of the funniest people I know! You always made me laugh when we worked together :) I am awed by your strength and courage during this journey. The way Mark writes about you is simply beautiful! Also, the love and support surrounding you is limitless!! I continue to pray for you and send you much love!!

Kelly Rothering

Mark and Debbie:

Some say you never know what's going on in someone's marriage, but I have figured out yours. Lots of love and tremendous respect and courage. I read your daily posts and think of you two all the time. I'm also the daughter of a breast cancer survivor. I sat with my mother when they told her the lump was malignant and watched her deal with the side effects of radiation. She got through all that and when she passed away in 2000, it was from something other than breast cancer. Hopefully, all of this will be behind you soon and this time next year will be very sweet. Keep up the fight.

Much love, Harriet Morganstein

Dear Debbie and Mark....

Mark, another beautifully written journal entry. I think you should save this and make a book for other cancer survivors, for the husbands that are taking this journey with their wives. You write from the heart. That is why you have captured everyone's attention. We love that you simply adore your Debbie, we treasure that you know and feel that she will be back to her old self. I think she will be even better than that.

Gina Millstein

Every Day - It's a Gettin' Closer
Written May 28, 2012 6:43 a.m.

Today will tell the tale as to whether tomorrow is D-Day and the drains are removed. The levels are looking good, not much is draining now at all. We hope for the best to reach a major milestone on the road to recovery.

Debbie had a good day, though she didn't get a real chance to rest much, but it's 8 a.m. now and she's still sleeping, so that's a good thing. She's playing catch-up.

Many thanks to her sister, Alisa, who came over yesterday and accomplished more in 6+ hours than I could in two days.

Let's hope this Memorial Day brings Deb the promise of freedom. D-Day Tuesday? We'll see. Thanks for caring,

Mark

Almost There, but Humbled
Written May 28, 2012 9:41 p.m.

As of tonight, it seems we are on the cusp of the next stage of our journey, drain-free. The levels of the drains at tonight's reading, combined with this morning's measurements, are where they need to be for the doctors to remove them tomorrow at our 9:30 a.m. appointment. They need to be gone. Deb started bleeding today from the site where the drain enters her body, then one of the plastic bubbles leaked out on her shorts later in the day. It's enough already. Time for them to go, and what a good day it would be. In fact, if the pain of the drain removal is not too great, the expectation is they will even inject 100cc of saline into her expanders, the first real step of reconstruction since the surgery 20 days ago. Keep hope alive.

I wasn't going to update again since this morning, but I wanted to put some thoughts down, and this is the place I put them. My apologies for wearing my emotions not just on my sleeve, but on my whole body, these past few months, but you can't believe how cathartic it is to keep a journal. I meant it as a place for updates en masse, but I don't have the time to write updates and keep a separate diary, so this is where I come to reflect and remember. In the end, I will print all of these pages out and save them. I don't want to go back—just not forget— the small things, the little moments that mean as much or more as the big picture.

With that in mind... today was one of those moments. It happened again. Debbie said something to me for which my response was silence.

I've spent large chunks of the past two days during this holiday weekend pressure washing the deck, porch, and stairs. We have an outside deck and a screened-in porch. Halfway through cleaning the porch today, I had to move a giant potted plant which sits on a tall stand. As I slid it across the decking, it caught on a seam and fell over, crashing to the ground. The pot smashed, the flowers got crushed, and there was potting soil everywhere. After cleaning it all up and finishing the project, I went inside to see how Deb was doing. I told her I had finished up, but there was a casualty—this beautiful large pot with the gorgeous flowers was history.

Old-world Debbie, she would have been upset; that pot is a large part of the porch decoration, and I probably would have been ordered to head out looking for a new one. New-world Debbie, she barely had anything to say about it, almost as if it never happened. Old-world, that would have been a focal point of our day. New world, it barely got a response. I said, "Since what we have been through, I can tell the little things don't bother you as much." She replied, "I've been humbled."

Humbled! So how do you respond? I didn't have a response, except for a half-smile and a nod—and the feeling I just wanted to wrap my arms around her and hold her tight and tell her how sorry I am. It's not fair for her to feel that way, because it's not her fault. Definition of humble: marked by meekness or modesty in behavior, attitude, or spirit. That's the one thing I don't want to have happen here—can't let the cancer battle crush her spirit, confidence, or zest for life. For me, the whole experience has re-awakened my focus on the positives in life—paying attention to the silver lining, giving of yourself, but not giving in, making a difference. Attitude is everything. These are all things I have strived to keep import-ant these past 10+ years that I have been self-employed. If not, you fail. But for Deb, her confidence, great sense of humor, her willingness to laugh at herself, her ability to call me out when I've gone too far, are all things I treasure about her. She has already sacrificed enough—can't let post-cancer "capture" her spirit. I won't let it.

There's a transition taking place here. As the physical pain and pressure begin to subside just a bit, it's the emotional side that starts to take center stage, if even in small doses. Still, I believe the next phase will be to keep it all in check. The physical part is easy to see—it's right out in front. But the emotional part is buried, either deep, or just below the surface. I think that will depend on the day or the environment we are in. Don't know when a word or an action might bring an emotional response. Whatever the challenge, I plan on being there and doing my best to make it better.

When I went to the garden center late today to replace the flowers and the pot (my idea, not Debbie's), I pulled up next to a Jeep that had a great saying printed on the wrapping of the spare tire. It read: "One Life, Live It."

We're all in.

Thanks for caring,

Mark

Freedom!

Written May 29, 2012 9:43 a.m.

D-Day. Mission Accomplished. They're out!! Drain-Free. Time to turn the page—more information and final post later.

Thanks for caring,

Mark

Winners: The Final Post

Written May 29, 2012 9:47 p.m.

Winners. It goes without saying, we feel like that now. The good day had two great "bookends"—Debbie getting her drains removed and then Emily's softball team, the one I co-manage, winning their softball game with the storm clouds rolling in and just one of the best damn double plays you'll ever see to finish a game.

Deb first. She was scared this morning, scared that pulling out the drains was going to hurt. From what she had read, it was time to double-up on the pain pills. But it wasn't so bad. At our appointment, Meg, our PA, warned her it would feel a little "wormy," but that would be about it. She was right. Deb said it felt like a worm being pulled out of her side. No pain... just gain. The gain I could see was the sense of relief on her face, dramatic relief, that this part was over. I could feel it, too. I said it before, the drains were like the umbilical cord that kept you tethered to the hospital, tethered to the surgery, tethered to the memory of that day, tethered to the remnants of what cancer did to her. Watching them get thrown in the trash was nirvana. Good-bye. Adios. Get the F*ck Out.

The ride home was like a new day. Though, just like this journey, there's always something that steals a little bit of the joy. Deb took that pain pill before the appointment, just in case. And now as we stopped at Santoni's for some food, she felt dizzy and had to get back in the car. We went home, and she got in bed for a nap. I was going to go to work. But my place was here, until she was ready to get up or our friends came by to bring her lunch. By noon, when I was ready to go, lunch and the girls arrived and Debbie was much better. Much, much better. And why shouldn't she be... a chapter closes and now a new one begins. It's the other reason I need to stop the daily postings. Time. More on that in a moment.

I forgot to mention that after they pulled the drains, they also filled the breasts with 50cc of saline, on each side. Meg, the PA, said it would start to round them out a bit at the bottom, and it did. I can already see when all is complete (and not that they weren't before), but these will be some spectacular Ta-Ta's. Ba ba booey.

Debbie will get injected every week for the next two months, until she gives the doctors the sign—"No Mas." By the end of July, that part will be over. We then wait two months more, and October, October 3rd to be exact, will be the second surgery to pull out the expanders and put in the implants.

Game, set, match. It will be outpatient surgery, but still a 1-2 week recovery. We leave for Vancouver on October 28th on a trip I earned through work, so we wanted it wrapped up by then. It will all be good. Taking Deb and her new "friends" international, baby.

Speaking of babies. How 'bout my baby's team, the Gators?! Down by three runs to the Terps in the top of the 4th inning, and with huge black storm clouds rolling in and the wind whipping up, my girls came from behind, scoring three runs and winning the game 7-5. My girls... winners!!

We're all winners. All of us. Every day you get up and breathe fresh air, you're winning. Every day a gift. Every day an adventure. Every day something unexpected. Good. Bad. Ugly. Funny. Heart stopping. Breathtaking. It's just life.

Life threw us a curveball, and we managed a big hit. We didn't strike out, not this time. Our at-bat was a courageous one. Much more so for the hitter, my wife, who stood in the batter's box and fouled off pitch after pitch, after pitch, until she finally decided to lay down a bunt. A sacrifice. Debbie's sacrifice. She took one for the team. Man, it hurts to say that. But it's true. I couldn't do it for her, though so many times I wished I could. All I could do was coach—offer support, offer encouragement, show love, compassion, and tell her we're gonna win this game. We did. This time. I'm not stupid enough to think that everything in life will be smooth sailing here on out. It's life. How does that saying go—if it was easy, everyone would do it. And everything would be perfect. It's not. Life ain't always beautiful. It wasn't meant to be. But what can be as close to perfect as possible is the way you choose to view what happens. Always expect the best, be positive, have a great attitude, smile, laugh, dream, plan, and be damn ready, so if the worst happens, you don't let it beat you down. And don't worry how you fell, focus on how you are going to get back up.

Winners. We feel like winners because everyone around us made us feel that way, and we can't thank you enough. There would never be enough room to express how we truly feel about everyone who has been there for us. The thank yous fall short, but it's all we've got. Just know, we'll be there for you, in thought, in prayer, in action. It's time to turn the page. Time to get back to life's most important job full-time—raising our daughters, Sophie and Emily. We gave life to them, and they are life's ultimate gift. Every day you get to keep unwrapping them and see what's inside that box. They never cease to amaze me. And why shouldn't they, they were born from the most amazing woman I have ever met... Debbie, my wife.

There's a new country song by Josh Turner that pretty much sums up why these postings need to stop. It's called "Time is Love." Search for it on YouTube if you want to give it a look and a listen. And from the bottom of my heart, thanks for listening to me.

And for one final time, thanks for caring.

Mark

Never Say Never Again
Written June 1, 2012 9:58 p.m.

With apologies to Sean Connery and the movie I referenced in the title, I'm back with the journal. There are a couple of reasons:

First, though we are in the recovery stage (drain-free), the journey is not over, far from it, and if I want to remember it and be able to reflect on it, or share it down the road, I need to keep going. Second reason—time. I've learned it takes less time to type an update than to answer the Facebook messages, the e-mails, texts, inquiries, or the face-to-face questions about

"How's Deb doing, what's the latest?" Third reason, just like Richard Gere in *Officer and a Gentleman*... "I've got no place to go!" I'm not going to write it all down (I can't read what I scribble). I'm not going to dictate it, cause then I would have to transfer it to written word. I'm not going to do it on some Microsoft Word document; it's too vanilla. Caringbridge is where I started, and it's the best place to update what's happening and record my thoughts and feelings so I don't forget. There will NOT be daily updates, just when it seems appropriate.

It's all about Deb, anyway. It might be my journal, but it's her story being written. I decided the story should define the appropriate ending, not the historian who is recording it. I was abusing my power by shutting it down completely.

So, the story continues. Debbie is doing much better. I knew back on Tuesday when the drains came out that the healing process would accelerate, and it has—maybe simply just because she feels better about things—the ball(s) and chain(s) are gone. Deb still gets tired easily, and there is still pain and soreness, plenty of it to be exact. But there's an overall feeling that we are over a huge hump. The sites where the drains entered Deb's body are healing, though one might be "slightly" infected, but no worse than if you had a small cut and it didn't heal right away. Otherwise, the areas where those plastic snakes with the bulbous heads once hung are now marked by only two small band-aids. Hallelujah and pass the hat.

Debbie even managed to make it to the Zac Brown Band Concert at Merriweather on Thursday night. Her health and demeanor compared to just 10 days earlier, when I literally had to hold her up at times to make it through the crowd at the Lady Antebellum concert, was like night and day. This time, she could clap and even raise her arms a bit. Just like Zac Brown sings. all she needed was to put "her toes in the water and her ass in the sand..." and all would have been well with the world. It was a good time.

There is an underlying fear, however. We have our post-op appointment with Dr. Friedman on June 13th, and Debbie is worried, not so much about that, but about what comes next. Dr. Friedman will recommend an oncologist for us to visit. Though Friedman believes no further treatment will be necessary, he will still defer to the decision of the oncologist. Deb has read that if a blood test is conducted and doesn't show the proper results, she could still face the possibility of chemotherapy. We'll see. In my heart, I don't believe so, but you can be damn sure if one doctor recommends it, we will be seeking a second opinion.

All in all, it's just good to have Debbie making a comeback. She even got behind the wheel of the car today for a few short trips around town. She still gets tired very easily, but she is doing a few "chores" (though I have told her not to), and it's great to have her at the dinner table with me and the girls.

Tonight, we all watched a movie together. Debbie reserved *The Vow* at Redbox, and I picked it up on my way home from work. I know, it's a chick flick. The deal is: I live with 3 of them!! Until you have done that, don't judge. You either adapt or get out. Besides, if it's a good movie, good story, I really don't care.

Actually, in the movie there were a couple of great lines, mainly the marriage vow spoken by Channing Tatum to Rachel McAdams, his movie wife:

"I vow to seriously love you, in all your forms, now and forever. I promise to never forget that this is a once in a lifetime love."

To my wife, Debbie... I vow the same.

Thanks for caring,

Mark

Guestbook Entries:

Dear Mark & Debbie,

Reading your heart-felt entries today has made me feel so many emotions. I am so happy her ordeal is about over—I am sad to read what you have all gone through so far. But mainly, I am heartened, to see God at work, and to see light at the end of the tunnel... Instead of asking, "Why did this happen," I find myself asking, "How does a couple cope with things when something like this happens?" But, Mark, you have always been very positive, meeting the world with a smile, and this proves attitude plays as big a role as the doctors, the hospital, and the medicines. I will keep praying for you, and thank you for sharing this private story will all of us "nose-y" readers on line...

Love to you, and Debbie, and your children.

Brenda Carl

Debbie, you are a warrior and an inspiration to all. Your girls are so lucky to have such a brave mama!!!

And Mark, for your girls to see how you are caring for and talking about their mother the way you are, I can't imagine them having a better role model in either of you.

You both are such amazing people. Every time I sit reading Mark's newest addition, I think that there had to be a silver lining to such a situation than this must be it. They are truly blessed.

xoxo Jan Silhavy

Please send my love to all of those strong women in your life. They are all very special. Continue enjoying each and every day you have together. Thanks so much for the updates.

Arlene Scherr

Weekend Wrap

Written June 3, 2012 9:50 p.m.

Debbie's weekend:

Going for a long walk Saturday morning—*Check.*

Watching Sophie play soccer on Saturday—*Check.*

Crabs and shrimp with the neighbors Saturday night—*Check.*

Hanging out on the porch Sunday afternoon w/friends—*Check.*

Taking a long walk on Sunday—*Check.*

Heating up dinner on Sunday—*Check.*

Helping with the laundry all weekend—*Check.*

Doing too much this weekend and now sore as sh*t—*Checkmate.*

Thanks for caring,

Mark

Battling

Written June 5, 2012 10:22 p.m.

The new routine begins. The next chapter of the recovery continues. Today was "injection day." We'll have one of these every week until the end of July. Saline is injected into each breast (this week 50cc in each) to expand the skin pockets and create the size Deb will want when all is said and done. Meg, the PA, said since the drains had been removed, the right breast also had some fluid backup, but she expected Debbie's body to absorb it. Nothing to be worried about. I'm sure the medical professionals are right, but famous last words... pardon the skepticism, but we've heard that way too much over the past few months.

This was the first appointment where I did not go. It's not easy to get to every single injection Debbie will have over the next two months, but I thank Lisa for taking Deb today. She can't and should not go by herself. It may not be dangerous, but emotionally, who needs to handle all of this alone?

It is still a battle. It's easy to say the "worst is over" and maybe it is. But for Deb, between being tired a lot and the pain AFTER the injection, it ain't easy. The expanders really hurt Debbie. She made the comment tonight that they hurt bad enough she wanted to take them out and just be "flat." Strong statement, but my girl doesn't give up. I expect she'll tough it out; she always does. More pain pills, please.

Speaking of battles, there was one that created a nice diversion for Deb (and I) tonight. Emily's softball team, the Gators (the one I co-manage), won game one of their tournament. Emily pitched the first inning and got out of a bases-loaded jam when she fielded a ball hit just short of the pitcher and threw a strike to third base to get the third out of the inning. She only gave up one run. Way to battle back, Emily. A few hours later, the Orioles battled the BoSox and came back three times to win the game. A day of battles.

A war has been won here for Deb, but the fallout will continue for some time to come. War has its casualties, sacrifices, and heroes. All were and are present these past few months. Prior to surgery, our war was fought with a game plan in mind, but the outcome in doubt; now, we fight every day with a strategy and a fairly predictable end (complete reconstruction). But the daily battle to get there has its own share of surprises, twists, and turns. You can't ever expect a day to be completely "normal." Though how many days in life are?

They are good, bad, or somewhere in between. It's not easy for Debbie. For me, maybe my years of being self-employed have helped. You get used to the daily rollercoaster ride of the highs and lows, so you never let either one get a hold of you; you stay planted firmly in the middle... with a positive attitude and always keep moving forward. That's where we are... and you can never forget that it could be much worse.

Debbie showed me an article just the other day about a 36-year-old woman who got breast cancer and had to go through a mastectomy and then chemotherapy. The chemotherapy alone almost destroyed her marriage. It made her sick, depressed, emotional, tired, and crazy. I can't see how putting poison into your body on a regular basis could make you anything but. It sucks. We just watched the movie "50/50" last week, and it was the same story—although the guy survived, the chemo was the worst. F*ck Cancer. I feel for everyone who has to go through with those poison treatments. The fact that cancer can make you poison yourself just to try and live is one of the worst scenarios. It reminds me of my father-in-law, who also had to make the decision to undergo those treatments to battle esophageal cancer. In the end, I believe it cost him his life... making his body so weak he couldn't fight off infection after his surgery. Still to this day, it's an unthinkable outcome, an unimaginable loss. The chemo takes those most full of life, just like Jerry, and sucks out every last drop. F*ck it all. I don't even get satisfaction from typing F*ck—it goes too deep. (I only put the asterisk in so they don't shut down the web page.)

But back to today. It's doubtful Deb will face any more treatment. As I mentioned before, it will be up to the oncologist, but it's unlikely we will see him or her before July. We meet with Dr. Friedman next week, and he will then recommend someone. I'm actually anxious to meet again with Friedman. I want to hear, firsthand, his analysis of everything that happened so far. The recap will be worth it, because it all happened so fast. Probably for the best. I wish I could speed things up for Debbie right now and get her to the end of October when she and I take our trip to Vancouver... post-surgeries, post reconstruction, post hell. I asked her tonight, "So what do we do in Vancouver?" She said, "It's a beautiful city, and if we can't find anything to do, we can just stare at my new breasts."

I'm all in.

Thanks for caring,

Mark

The Song

Written June 7, 2012 5:49 a.m.

No need for many words. Had not listened to this song since the surgery. Last night, Debbie ASKED me to pull it up on You Tube.

It's Martina McBride's song: "Gonna Love You Through It."

The video does it justice. Needs to be part of the journal. You will have to wait out the :30 sec ad, but it's worth it.

(You can search for this song on YouTube.)

Thanks for caring,

Mark

Tributes

Written June 10, 2012 6:50 a.m.

A touching tribute yesterday from Jake Rosenbaum and part of his Bar Mitzvah project to honor Debbie and the battle she fought and sacrifice she made to rid herself of breast cancer. During his speech, Jake let everyone know how the entire

Reisterstown Baseball League wore pink bracelets for a game a few weeks back in honor of Deb. It brought Debbie to tears—knew it would—how could it not? We thank Jake for his amazing and heartfelt tribute to Debbie. We've known him since the day he was born, what a great kid, and his parents, Keith and Debbie, among our closest friends... the family you meet along the way.

Debbie is doing better. But for all her strength, courage, and ability to handle the physical pain of the biopsy, surgery, and recovery, there is still the emotional balancing act, the day-to-day reminder of reality, and thoughts of the past, pre-cancer. Deb says she thinks she has handled it all pretty well—I view that as the understatement of the year. There are people we run into each and every day who can't believe she is out—at the store, at a concert, at a Bar Mitzvah, over at a neighbor's house for dinner. That's Debbie. I always knew once the drains were removed, so were the chains that seemed to tie her down... making her feel like she had to be home. She still gets tired often. Yesterday's Bar Mitzvah wiped her out for the afternoon, but she recovered to head down the street for a neighborhood get-together.

The week ahead will be a busy one with another injection Tuesday, a post-op appointment with Dr. Friedman on Wednesday, then off to the beach for a week of R & R on Saturday. Upon diagnosis back in April, we wondered if our annual family trip to the beach in June would happen. It's a tribute to the doctors who scheduled us in so quickly and performed two amazing surgeries, a tribute to our friends and family who have supported us every step of the way, and a tribute to the patient—my survivor—who has faced every trial and tribulation of the journey with a strong will and focus on getting up, getting out, and getting better. It's easy to take for granted the woman Debbie is—others might not be so strong, others might not still be able to laugh at the world and themselves, others might have never reached for and conquered the "goals" she has accomplished already. My wife continues to amaze me every day.

I can only hope this journal, in its entirety, will one day be a fitting tribute to her beautiful spirit and a heartfelt reminder of our incredible journey together. Debbie deserves it. The best is yet to come.

Thanks for caring,

Mark

The Process and the Payoff

Written June 13, 2012 11:20 p.m.

"It's a process." Pretty black and white, huh? That's the takeaway I had from this morning, when we visited Dr. Friedman for Debbie's post-op appointment and he said the above statement. Okay. He's right. Well, kind of.

We did more this morning by 10 a.m. than most former cancer patients do all day. Our 8:30 a.m. appointment with Dr. Friedman went pretty well; he and his assistant examined Debbie and said things look good. And they will only get better. After the examination, we stepped into his office to hear the results one more time. Two very small cancerous tumors, 3mm or less, all gone. Only in the right breast, nothing in the left breast. So what now? An appointment with an oncologist one floor below Friedman's office. Friedman believes nothing more needs to be done in terms of "follow up" post-cancer care. Debbie asked him about chemotherapy. "Chemo?" he said. "If that is recommended, call me and we will get a second opinion." So what about Tamoxifen? Friedman says there is only about a 5% chance cancer could show up again. If you take Tamoxifen, the odds are reduced by about 1%. If that's the case, why try it? However, we will first hear the recommendation, if any, from the oncologist when we meet with him in two weeks.

Setting the oncologist appointment was enough for me. Just one floor below Dr. Friedman's office—the fourth floor—is the Cancer Treatment Center. Wow. As positive as the experience you feel visiting Dr. Friedman and Dr. Chang (the plastic surgeon)—their offices are warm and welcoming—in contrast to the treatment center, it's shocking. It was darker, and there was this hum coming from the ceiling and the air conditioning unit that made it hard to hear, or think, or feel anything else but gloom and doom. I couldn't get out of there fast enough. I feel for all those who must go there on a daily, or semi-regular, basis. My prayers are with you. Heal fast, my friends.

We also paid a visit to the Breast Shoppe, where Debbie was fitted with some special silicone bras and halter tops. The bras make it look almost like nothing has happened—pretty amazing, except when you are living "the process." Debbie had to undress three different times today in the span of 90 minutes—Dr. Friedman, Dr. Chang, the Breast Shoppe. She spent her morning taking her clothes off and putting them back on... it was a routine that you wish could stop, not because I think anything looks wrong, but because it's just enough. She's not saying that, I am. "It's a process." F*ckin right, it's a process. Easy to say, a little different when you are living it. The fact that I'm up at 11:30 p.m. doing an update confirms the process... I need to vent, to remember, to break down the details in a way that I won't forget.

Debbie also got another injection, 50cc of saline in each breast, the most that Meg, the PA, feels Deb should have, since she complains of being sore from the injections. And her back is giving her a lot of trouble, as well. Some medicine and possibly some PT should help make things better.

And speaking of better, as strange as the day began, it ended just the opposite, at least for me. I got to spend time with Marty, one of my favorite people and the person who has always been a big brother to me. Thanks, bro, always good to see you and to catch up. Nice to know you are always there. And great to see Sharon and their daughter, Savannah. On the drive home tonight, thinking of Savannah brought a big smile to my face—not just because of the incredible person she has become (I've known her since she was a baby), but she reminds me, as do my own children, of how life has a way of bringing you moments that make you stop, stare, and appreciate a beautiful miracle every now and then. You realize that somehow everything will be okay. That this "process" for Debbie, which indeed has had its own miracle, will eventually lead to peace and happiness. That no matter what, if you have people to count on, people who love you and you love back, life will just keep on going.

For Debbie, that's the gift she's been given. Life. Actually, for those who love her, that's the gift she's already given us—the greatest gift of all. Thanks for being our hero. The payoff will be worth the fight... and then some. I promise.

Thanks for caring,

Mark

Father's Day, Fun, and Fractures

Written June 18, 2012 10:40 a.m.

Father's Day. Only four words to describe it: "I can't go there." I mean do you REALLY want me to pour my heart out on THIS Father's Day and what it means to me? Just can't go there.

Unfortunately, where I should not have gone was the beach yesterday, as I fractured my fibula (non-displaced), while playing pop-flies with the girls. The vacation is far from over, but it certainly curtails one of my most important responsibilities, which is helping to care for Debbie. Now, we will both be recovering together. Though mine is miniscule compared to hers... and I hope to have a walking boot by today to make getting around much easier.

Deb is better, but still gets tired, can't lift heavy objects, still experiences pain—in fact, last night she said it felt like she was having a heart attack—the pain was shooting and severe in her chest. But she rebounded, as my hero always does. I felt the spot where her expander pad sticks out... it is hard and obtrusive, you can imagine not a fun object to have in your chest and pushing on your muscles.

So here we are at the beach for year 13 of our annual family tradition with the Cummins' and my mother-in-law and her friend, Lloyd. 10 of us in all. If you had told me on April 13th, when Deb was diagnosed, that we'd be on the beach relaxing in the sun yesterday—with Deb looking so great—I would have told you I hoped we'd make it—that it's 50/50.

The journey now enters its "resting phase," as we enjoy a summer vacation with family. About 65 days since the world flipped for us—less than 40 days since we flipped cancer "the bird" with a surgery to knock out the bastard, and 20 days since the doctors popped out the f*cking drains, Deb was sitting on a beach chair, resting easy, listening to music. Let's give credit where credit is due, my survivor is one strong, beautiful woman. The pot of gold is still months away—completion of the reconstruction—but at least now you can see the rainbow breaking through the clouds.

Sitting on the beach, looking out at the ocean, which seems to go on forever, and glancing over at my survivor on the chair next to mine, with her eyes closed, resting at ease, might just be the best, most blessed place to be. If you can't get even a little humbled, or spiritual, looking out at the never-ending Atlantic Ocean on a summer day, you need to check your life card at the door. It's time to step off the planet.

Like I said, Father's Day—and its meaning to me this year—I can't write that essay, because salt water doesn't mix well with the computer keys. But as we were driving to our beach destination on Saturday, with my survivor, Debbie, asleep in the passenger seat, and my two miracles, Sophie and Emily, asleep in the back seat, I took a glance in my rearview mirror. Far back on the road behind me, I could still see the hazy memories of the early parts of the journey—the doctor appointments, procedures, diagnosis, surgery, drains, utter exhaustion, pain-filled days, and sleepless nights. But we are picking up speed along the road and putting even greater distance between us and the event that tried to detour our lives for good. The road before me says Yield, instead of Stop. The lights are turning green, one by one. Life is moving forward. We are not in cruise control just yet—and maybe we'll never be there completely— but we're starting to coast just a little.

There was a song on the radio as I glanced at all my girls, resting peacefully on the drive to the beach: "Me and You" by Kenny Chesney. Perfect.

(You can search for this song on YouTube.)

Thanks for caring,

Mark

Pain: Front to Back
Written June 24, 2012 11:21 a.m.

The circle of pain. A little more than six weeks since Deb's surgery, and for more than almost two weeks now she has been complaining of back pain. It's a combination of things: the muscle expander pads, sleeping on her back a lot, making adjustments because of the pain up front, and I have to believe the stress she feels sometimes from the whole darn experience.

Deb has already had one visit to physical therapy and a massage to try and get a handle on the new "consequence" of the double mastectomy, the expander pads, and the injections of saline. Certain exercises, the massage, only seem to provide a band-aid for the newest trouble spots. You have a feeling it's going to be like this for some time, at least until the injections stop at the end of July. Still, what's the line you hear so often... "It could be much worse." True. Still doesn't make you feel the pain any less.

We just wrapped up a week at the beach for family vacation. Went well, though my fractured fibula didn't make things any better. I still can't bear weight, but what I hate is for Debbie to bear any more weight, taking care of me. The last thing I wanted was for her to do more than she should. Until I can walk on two feet, unfortunately, there are not a lot of alternatives.

I have to say Deb looked great in her bathing suits, though she said, especially on our last beach day, how painful the suits were on her expander pads. Thought the drains were a bitch—and they were—more than a bitch—these expander pads apparently aren't a party, either. In fact, last night, Deb thought there might be a lump at the site where the drains used to be. I took a look and felt the area. The word lump is not what you want to hear, but there wasn't one, it was just the point of one of the pads sticking out. What fun.

The week ahead will be an interesting one. I get to see the ortho surgeon—our cousin, Dr. Zooker—to check out what the prognosis is on the left leg. Debbie has two appointments, back to back on Tuesday. Up first is our meeting with Dr. Chang, the plastic surgeon, for the first time since the surgery. I am interested to hear his thoughts. Then, immediately following that appointment, the "moment of truth" meeting with the oncologist, Dr. Riseberg. It might be Debbie's biggest fear right now. We will discuss the cancer surgery, the cancer itself, the prognosis and what, if any, follow-up treatment would be necessary. It's that baby elephant in the room—the cancer is gone, but must anything be done to make sure nothing "leaked" out? The lymph nodes were clear, but did any micro-cells make their way somewhere else in Debbie's body?

At most, if anything, it would be Tamoxifen. But the surgeon told us that in Debbie's case taking Tamoxifen might change the odds by about 1% that cancer might resurface somewhere. Is it worth taking it, is it worth the side effects, would there be side effects? Questions still yet to be answered. The surgeon said the oncologist would know best how to explain and discuss the options. Fair enough. We hope for the best.

Hope. Sometimes, it's all you can do.

Thanks for caring,

Mark

As Good as It Gets

Written June 26, 2012 9:49 p.m.

So what more could you want? No need to bury the lead, I'm going to explain it right now. The oncologist, Dr. Riseberg, said he wouldn't recommend any more treatment. Nothing. Nada. Zilch.

Since April 13th when the diagnosis was official, that moment today in the oncologist's office was the closest I came to tearing up in front of one of the docs. I had to push back the lump in my throat as I listened to the doctor, THE doctor, the one who faces the beast every day and tries to defeat it, tell us that, based on his expert opinion, less is more.

Based on the pathology results, the fact the cancer was caught early, the fact that the tumors were small, Tamoxifen would have been the only consideration, anyway. Not chemotherapy, not radiation, not any alternative treatments. And the issue with Tamoxifen is this—the small benefit you might gain, and we're talking maybe a 1% differential between taking it and not taking it, is canceled out by the risks. There is a slight risk for those who take Tamoxifen of blood clots or stroke! So the risk vs. reward here isn't worth it. Imagine having a stroke because you took a medication you really didn't need in the first place. That would REALLY suck.

Now understand this is how it all went down and this is my perspective. Debbie's thoughts were a little more on the emotional side. After hearing what the doctor said, she replied she was "comfortable" with his recommendation of doing nothing. But she took notes when he spoke, and she still wanted to know what the window was, should she freak out and decide she wanted to do everything she possibly could to make sure the cancer would never return. The risk of cancer returning locally is as close to zero as you can get. Could there be micro-cells? The oncologist said it's doubtful. Only a few percent chance, and again Tamoxifen would only change that by 1%, if that. The window for Debbie to change her mind is about 3 months.

Bottom line: we are not doing anything. The text I sent to a few of my friends today: "Oncologist confirmed it for us—nothing else needed. All clear. Deb should go live her life." I think that pretty much sums it up. There may be some genetic testing down the road, just to make sure Debbie is not carrying some mutated gene that she could pass to our daughters. Again, I believe that not to be the case. It just happened—Debbie got breast cancer, she made the right call with a double mastectomy (the oncologist confirmed that fact today, especially with her family history), and the pathology showed it's all gone. The reconstruction continues, but besides that—let's say it once and for all—F*CK THE CANCER.

A little retrospective—today's appointments didn't go exactly as planned. Deb was supposed to meet with the plastic surgeon, Dr. Chang, and get more saline injections into the breasts and then go downstairs and meet with the oncologist, but it didn't go down like that. Chang was running way behind, so we were forced to have the meeting with Dr. Riseberg, the oncologist first, then come back upstairs for the injections. And ya know what? It worked out perfectly, because after getting the good news, it made the injection appointment more pleasant, if that's the right word. It was like somebody blew a big gray cloud right out of the room. In fact, Deb went for double the amount of the injection today, 100cc into each breast. There may only need to be two or three injections more before she is at the size she desires.

And she looks great. I can't say that enough. Nor can anyone else. But it's not always other people's opinions that matter. Deb has told me repeatedly over the past few days she hates the way she looks. All I can do is reassure her that she looks fantastic. I know that it's the emotional side of this journey coming out in fits and starts. Debbie has been so damn good at not being upset, at keeping herself in check, at being as close to the perfect patient as possible, that at some point there has to be a crack in the armor. She can't possibly escape from the emotional toll these procedures, one by one, are having on her. Love and support—which have been over the top—and her own incredible determination and fighting spirit have their breaking point. It was in grand display this past weekend, when this bitch cashier at the Giant made Debbie put all the items back in her cart when Deb missed the "12 items only" sign at the register. When Deb told the woman she was so sorry and it was her first time at the grocery store since her surgery, the cashier couldn't care less and watched Deb take her items, one by one, from the belt and put them back in her cart and then find a new, long line to stand in. Debbie cried for hours after that incident. It wasn't the fact she messed up; it was the fact the cashier showed so little compassion, supposedly even smirking as Debbie struggled to replace her grocery items in the cart. I wasn't on hand for the incident, only the aftermath. It's part of the emotions Deb has kept in check—leaking out—but this time the flood gates opened.

Debbie is also not having an easy time with me, either. Since fracturing my fibula on Father's Day, it has not been a picnic. I won't be able to bear weight on the f*cker for five more weeks and need a good bit of assistance around the house. It was the last thing I ever wanted to have happen. I don't want to burden someone who had to carry the burden so recently, but we'll get through it—and I just picked up a roll-a-bout to help me move quicker around the house and be able to carry items at the same time. If it seems like an eternity since we went through cancer surgery—and it does—this temporary fracture will heal and I'll be back to walking before you know it.

And speaking of healing... that's what it feels like tonight. After a somewhat tense and emotional day, it feels like we've crossed over to the other side—officially. It feels even more complete than the day Dr. Friedman called to give us the pathology results following surgery, or the day we said adios to the dreaded drains. The diagnosis, while shocking, was attended to quickly, the surgery was a resounding success, the initial recovery, while challenging and scary at times, reached its major milestone when the drains were removed, and the reconstruction, which brings with it some new consequences, including back pain, is for the most part coming along about as well as can be expected. I'll say it again, because it bears repeating—Debbie looks great. More beautiful than ever, if that's possible.

My bride, my survivor, my hero, is one in a million—she is also one of millions who battle the same evil. Her fight has been a strong and swift one, and with very, very positive results. Too many don't get the good news—we feel for them, we pray for them, we hope that one day, and one day soon, there won't need to be a fight at all. One day, we'll find the cure.

But for now, we live out the life we have been given, with all its imperfections and challenges, but much joy—too much to mention. Today was a day of joy. I think Dr. Riseberg put it best when he said, "The cancer is not a blessing by any means, but the outcome is about as good as it gets."

Amen.

Thanks for caring,

Mark

(Debbie's) Independence Day!!
Written July 4, 2012 9:50 a.m.

So is it that milestones keep happening right around the holidays, or can I somehow find a way to bridge the connection of meaning between steps along the journey and significant days on the calendar? Whatever, another big, big moment in this next chapter of the recovery—the final "fill." The fill—the injection of saline into each breast, the weekly appointment to expand the breasts to the point where Deb said "I'm done"— that day has happened.

On the eve of Independence Day, Deb had what turned out to be her final fill. Dr. Chang injected 50cc of saline into each breast and confirmed with Debbie that if she wanted to be the size of a "small C" in breast measurement, she's there. So no more injections. Now we sit it out for two months. It's all good news. And because of the early arrival at the finish line, we were able to bump up the date of the next surgery to September 19th, instead of our original scheduled date of October 3rd. During the second surgery, the expanders will be removed and the silicone implants will be placed in each breast, size "C." The recovery on that second surgery, which is outpatient (like Deb joked, the first surgery was nearly outpatient as fast as they force you out of the hospital), will require a 1-2 week recovery time. But NO drains. Ready to join hands with anyone who wants to and sing "Hallelujah" on that one! We will meet with Dr. Chang a few days before surgery to outline the process and what to expect during the recovery phase. Minor surgery? Every surgery is minor, until it happens to you.

Gotta admit I'm jealous. I wasn't there yesterday. We thought we'd have two more injections, so I was planning on being there for the final one next week. Thanks to Jill and Marni for taking Deb to the appointment, but had I known we were wrapping it all up, I would have been there, as well. When Deb texted me "all done fills," I was excited and a bit saddened at the same time, because there was an important milestone I had missed. Those moments along the journey are the ones where you post the mile marker and look back when it's all over to say "remember when." Look, there will be many more to come, and many more have passed, but still it hurt just a bit.

So the 4th of July brings with it true independence for Debbie. The first day of a two-month respite—free from doctors, needles, injections, surgeries, waiting for final reports from oncologists, and wondering when the "fills" would be enough. Just over 80 days since diagnosis and this is where we are. Talk about an eventful three months of life. Now there's time to rest before the implants—gear up for the next chapter of the journey—cancer free and all filled up! And filled up in more ways than one, with thanks, love, and gratitude that all will be okay in the end. I heard Debbie say out loud what I had put in writing several times before, what the breast surgeon, the plastic surgeon, and the oncologist had confirmed—the sacrifice was worth it. It could have been much worse; having had to go through a double mastectomy to conquer the beast, there could have been many, many other consequences.

I believe the true emotional toll has yet to be determined, or even to completely surface, but we'll face it as it comes. Certainly, there is the huge sense of relief and gratefulness for the best outcome possible. Couldn't be more proud of the woman

I married and how she has carried herself throughout the ordeal. A true hero.

So now it's time to enjoy the holiday. Time for a signed "declaration" of R & R. Happy Birthday America and Happy Independence Day for Deb.

Thanks for caring,

Mark

Sixty Days
Written July 9, 2012 6:36 p.m.

It's just a number, but it's significant. 60.

60 seconds in a minute. 60 minutes in an hour. 60 days in a life.

July 10th marks 60 days since the surgery. 60 days Since Debbie was forced to give up a part of her being in order to end up being okay. I've often thought what stands out more, the diagnosis or the double mastectomy. One was going to happen no matter what you did, the latter took a conscious, brave, and in the end, logical decision to execute a life-altering event—a sacrifice that any woman can relate to, can empathize.

The physicality of the event is easy to document. You can look it up in any medical report dealing with breast cancer. The emotional journey is an uneven story yet to be finished, maybe ever. I can, and so can many others, tell Debbie time and time again how great she looks. I tell people all the time, "Just look at her, and tell me that you would have known the girl had breast cancer and a double mastectomy just two months ago." Impossible. The "fills" have her back to just about where she was before in breast size, and she looks just as stunning as ever, on the outside.

But spend a day in her soul and you would know a lot more. She doesn't talk a ton about it—she lets you know when she's hurting physically, when she's tired, when her back aches, when she has a headache, and when she's had enough for the day. She told me tonight just before she went out, and right after I told her how great she looked, how she "hates her body," how she "hates the extra skin near the breasts," how she "hates the scars from the drains." I hate that she has to feel any hate at all. I hate that I can't always wrap my head around what she is feeling inside and instead just want to wrap my arms around her and let her know how much she's loved.

I don't see many tears, but I can sense the hurt inside. I saw a picture online yesterday and copied it and sent it to Deb. It read, "People cry, not because they are weak. It's because they've been strong for too long." The strongest of concrete foundations are poured onto soft ground. There is always a weakness, and it's okay to let it show, it's okay to feel it. You can't run away from it; you can only kick the watering can down the road until it breaks and the floodgates open.

So many times, I wish Deb's dad was still here. He witnessed it all from somewhere, though, had he still been here, I believe it might have pained him more than anyone to watch his baby girl suffer. But in recovery, he would be the one to "shore Deb up," keep her laughing, and make sure she could "let go," as well.

60 days. I watched Debbie roller skate around the rink yesterday at Emily's birthday party, wondering just how we could have come so far in such a short time. I saw the look on her face, the joy of being free, of doing something that in all our minds takes you back to a time when you were much younger and things like cancer happened to other people, or you just didn't know enough to care.

It's a moment in time, still. But time never stands still. Maybe that's the hardest part of all of this—there is no "time" for

Deb to stop and be as thankful, as reflective, as joyful, or even to break down and have a good cry. Life moves too fast. You glance away, and the moment before is already in the rearview mirror. So you keep going, but without the "time" to really take it all in. So later, when something happens that triggers a memory, or pisses you off, or disappoints you, or makes you feel small... that's when it all catches up with you. That's when you realize what you've been through, or just maybe, if you're lucky, you can stop and revel in the fact that you accomplished so much since then.

60 days. Two months. More memories, more moments, more feelings than you can fit onto a page. Debbie is a different person, as am I. Stronger, better, different. We're still working through it together. The journey has a ways to go. Hand in hand, we'll make it.

Deb loves the Kelly Clarkson song "Stronger," and with good reason: It says what doesn't kill you makes you stronger and stand taller. My girl deserves to stand so tall she can reach the stars.

So pull one down, Deb, and make a wish... and let's hope it comes true.

Thanks for caring,

Mark

Genes and Screams
Written July 17, 2012 5:48 a.m.

Just past the three-month mark since diagnosis, more than two months since the surgery, and yesterday was a visit to Dr. Friedman's (the breast surgeon) assistant, Jean.

Debbie was most impressed with Jean and her knowledge of the situation. She knew "everything about everything" that has happened so far, even the family history. So while Jean said all looks good, the cancer is gone, the fills are complete, and everything is progressing as planned... there is still an open question. Is it in the genes?

My mother-in-law had the genetic testing some years back and all was clear. But, obviously, testing and medicine advance at lightning speed (thank G-d and let's hope health-care reform doesn't kill that spirit), and now there is more accurate testing—plus, because of the family history, Jean said we should get an answer once and for all to make sure Debbie isn't carrying any "mutated" genes, which would mean the ovaries would be the next to go!! A hysterectomy. On top of that, we have the health of two daughters to consider down the road.

Deb doesn't mess around. With that in mind, she booked an appointment with the genetic testing center at Mercy. So about a week before the surgery, we will have some initial blood work, then they will make a decision from there how to proceed for more testing. Talk about a hot, unsettling summer. I am staying on the positive side of this fence, though—what's done is done, and it's over.

Still every time you think it's over, a hint of doubt or some other concern seems to linger. Seems to be the way the journey goes. It's like trying to overcome the obstacle course in basic training. There's another challenge at every turn. We still, of course, have the second surgery planned for September 19th. The good news is Jean confirmed with Debbie that once those implants are in, things will feel much better all around. Good to hear, since Deb still has soreness in her chest and back, pretty much on a daily basis.

Also on a daily basis is the courage and strength Deb continues to demonstrate. It's a much calmer time overall, but like

I've mentioned before, the emotional side of everything, the wear and tear of constant ups and downs, take their toll. I've seen evidence in the past week—Debbie is not one to "mess with" right now. She is stronger, more confident, and a touch more aggressive than before. Just ask the Transit police officer who tried to stop us from getting to a certain parking lot at the concert at Merriweather Post the other night. He isn't planning any "Let's Celebrate Debbie" parades, I'm sure. She let him have it (verbally of course) when he tried to be a smart ass. There was no slow burn; Debbie gave him an immediate tongue lashing like I have rarely seen her do to someone. In a way, it was fun to watch—in another way, Deb is still letting it all out—but in small explosive doses, kind of like letting the steam out of the kettle, then capping it, then opening it, then capping it, then opening it. Eventually, it will all escape; I just hope I'm not in the way to get burned!!

It's okay, though. Lord knows, Deb deserves the opportunity to vent—give up a part of yourself and you've earned the right to give some back!! And speaking of giving, our continued thanks to those who continue to "give" every day in their unwavering support of all Deb has endured. It is amazing how many people come up to me and let me know that they still follow Debbie's progress every step of the way. The hard steps of the journey are softened by your feelings of love and compassion ... we can feel it. Believe me. And it will never, ever be forgotten.

Thanks for caring,

Mark

The Dog Days

Written August 3, 2012 11:28 a.m.

So it's not exactly the calm before the storm. It's more like my favorite Tom Petty song: "The Waiting is the Hardest Part." Surgery #2 is less than 40 days away. So what do you do? You hang around and wait. August and half of September will be spent biding our time until Debbie goes back under the knife. So while the last doctor visit was the last "tangible" thing that occurred along the journey, the more recent, calmer, less dramatic days are the times that the emotions start to seep out. The less you have going on, the more you start to think a little deeper about what has happened and how it's all affecting you.

I can see it in Debbie every day now. She continues to say how she hates the way she looks... yet she is more beautiful than ever. But I know what she is referring to. And I know how it is slowly taking its toll. It's like the slow drip of a faucet, every few minutes, or seconds, you hear or see the drop. And no matter how tight you turn the screw, it just keeps dripping, slow and steady. That's what is going on here... Deb lets it out a little at a time, disgust, anger, disappointment, fear, and sadness about what has been lost, about what has been sacrificed at a young age. Once in a while, that drip becomes a stream of water, of tears, of a slight breakdown in her mental and emotional fortitude. When the strongest of us finally crack, it comes out in waves.

But surgery #2, the implants, should bring redemption. We just got finished watching gymnast Jordan Wieber suffer her life's biggest disappointment and then come back to help her U.S. Gymnastics team win it all... beaming all the way. It's what I want for Deb. She's already a champion, she's already a winner, but she suffered a setback in life that was not of her own doing. And now it's time for the comeback, the realization of what can be, and the feeling of accomplishment for seeing it all the way through, with a smile on her face, at least for the rest of the world to see. The toughest competitors, the greatest champions, show composure to those watching them, in victory and in defeat. That's my girl. She is showing everyone how it's done, even on the days when she's "done." Done with putting on the best face possible and forcing herself to feel good about everything. I gotta say, though, I've learned over time, if you say it out loud, you believe it. The mere utterance of the words tricks your mind into believing it is real. Tell yourself you are happy and you look good enough, and you should start to accept it as fact. For Debbie, IT IS A FACT; she just needs to say it to herself again and again.

The dog days of August will be broken up with our girls returning from camp, another trip to the beach, and the hustle and bustle of getting ready for school to start again. Before you know it, Labor Day will be here and then the real countdown to implant surgery on September 19th. It will all be here, and it will all be over before you know it. Then another few weeks of recovery and getting used to the new breasts. We'll find out what Dr. Chang is really made of. Though I've got this feeling... they might not be real, but they will be spectacular!! Just like the person to whom they belong. My girl, my champion, Debbie.

Thanks for caring,

Mark

30 Days to Daylight; Thanks O's

Written August 19, 2012 11:03 p.m.

30 Days. September 19th will mean a new chapter, hopefully the start of the final chapter in the journey when Debbie goes back under the knife for the implants. And so we wait and count the days. Much has happened over the past few weeks—

time for fun with friends and family, the girls returning from camp, another trip to the beach—all a lot of fun.

There were also painful moments. Deb having to deal with my recovery from my ankle injury, which was a super-hot and super frustrating period of six weeks, nearly half the summer. All the while, Deb still dealing with the emotional ups and downs of where she is right at this moment. Most of the time, she's a trooper. Then there are the moments, like the one we shared in the Atlantic Ocean during our recent trip to Rehoboth, where she asked the question, half-joking, "Why did this happen to me?" How can you, how do you, answer? What do you say, what is appropriate? "Cause shit happens?" Not exactly the deepest of comebacks, but there really is no way to adequately come up with the right response. We all know the saying (or is it the book), "Why Bad Things Happen to Good People;" there's no rhyme or reason. Is it that the Lord above has a plan and wants to test your resolve? Maybe. Is it that it's just part of life, and challenges present themselves to everyone at one time or another? Maybe. Is it that it's just random, and there is just no answer? Probably. Deb deserves to ask the question, again and again, if she likes, but there will never be an answer that suits the situation. It's just not black and white.

Instead, it's best to focus on what makes you happy, take your mind off what comes next (though the next step should eventually make Deb happy), and look for inspiration all around us—in our children, in our family, from our friends, from the smallest wonders you rarely take time to appreciate, to the largest in-your-face moments that bring a smile to your face.

One of those moments happened a few weeks back, before Sophie and Emily returned from camp. One night, we hopped on the light rail and headed to Camden Yards for the Orioles game. I secured some prime seats, and we got to enjoy what we hadn't had a chance to do (or wanted to do since the O's have sucked for more than a decade) since we had kids. We got to go to an O's game together—just us—one of the things we most enjoyed, and one of the things we knew we had in common when we first met, our love for baseball, especially the Orioles. Though we lost, and I was on crutches at the time, it was still a great night. It took me back to those days when things were a bit simpler for us and the world was just a slightly different shade of happiness, without the worry of illness or recovery.

I have to say, thank you, Orioles, for this season. However it ends up, you have created a daily distraction that has been inspiring and heartwarming. The O's took off on a winning season in April, just as Debbie was diagnosed, and they have served as a tremendous distraction during all we have gone through. Funny how sports, which doesn't "really" matter in the big scheme of things, can matter so much when you need to be inspired, to get your heart racing and extract some much needed joy from that same heart.

And heart is where I will leave it. All out there in the open as we set forth on the final weeks and days of this chapter along the journey. The book has yet to be finished; we still have a ways to go. But my heart is where it needs to be, especially as I lay down for the night, next to the heart to which I have given mine. I love you, Debbie.

Thanks for caring,

Mark

Guestbook Entries:

Dearest Debbie,

After having just read the latest post to the journal, we just want you to know that we wonder all the time "Why you?" Maybe it is that we need to live each day to the fullest with our kids, our family, and our friends, and especially our Sophie and Emily. Honestly, since April, there has been such an awakening call for us to

take each day and realize how in a second, a minute,
an hour life can change so drastically. No matter what,
you have the right to wonder "Why me?" because we,
too, wonder "Why you?"

Since you are our special "daughter," we never want to
see anything happen to anyone we love so dearly. We
are just so happy that you, Mark, and the girls had a
blast in Rehoboth. No one deserved it more!

We love you always!

Bonnie and Robin Brodinsky (Mom & Dad)

Excited and Nervous

Written September 4, 2012 10:11 p.m.

No, the title of the journal entry has nothing to do with the Orioles being in 1st place (though ain't it grand?). It does have to do with Debbie, for the first time since that dark day back in April, saying the word "excited" when it has anything to do with this cancer thing—or post-cancer thing.

I debated on an update because we had a fairly important doctor appointment today, then I heard her say those words to her friend, Ellen, on the phone tonight. Excited? Yup, I heard right. Deb said she was "excited" that this will soon be over. Who wouldn't be? I think it was more like "excited, but still nervous." Still. It is the beginning of the end.

In two weeks—September 19th—my bride will go under the knife again for the breast implants. Silicone, small "C." No, not real, but sure to be spectacular, especially with the work being done by the talented Dr. Chang.

I was there for the pre-surgery appointment with Dr. Chang today. It's the same routine we have seemed to have gone through a thousand times now. Doc is running late. We get called back. Nurse tells Deb to get undressed and put on the gown. It's SSDA. Same shit, different appointment.

Doc says everything looks good. The pain will be "magnitudes less" than it was after the cancer and breast removal surgery back in May. And best of all—no drains!! Some pain, no drain. Silver lining. The surgery will take about 90 minutes. We need to be there two hours early, just about 8 a.m. that day. Then post-surgery is two hours in recovery. The day will start early and end late. A long day.

But this time, there's a payoff. I guess that's the right word. Debbie will have perfectly shaped silicone implants, in the place where just a few months ago there was an unwelcome invader trying to grow and take her down. But Deb fought back, with a vengeance, a resolve, and a strength that few can muster. My hero is one strong woman.

And woman she is. She said something to me the other day on a drive home from dinner, "Did it still seem surreal?" Can I (me) believe it all really happened? Ah, another think-about-it-too-much and choke-back-the-tears moment. Just love 'em. Can't get enough. So I answer: I tell her I still can't believe it. I still think it's crazy she had to have her breasts removed. That she had to give up a part of what defines a woman.

But I owe Debbie an apology. I was dead wrong. It's what helps define a female, not a woman. The female simply has those "other" body parts, including the breasts; it's just part of biology. They don't define a woman. A woman is defined by what's in her soul, how others view her in their heart, and in the eyes of the two miracles that are asleep just down the hall from us, our daughters. Maybe more so than the love I hold inside for Deb, she as a woman is defined by looking into the eyes of Sophie and Emily and the way they look at her. All beautiful.

Breasts be damned. They're simply cosmetic accoutrements to the person to whom they belong, but they don't make her a woman. I wouldn't love her any less, nor would her girls look upon her as anything but their devoted, loving Mom, had she decided against reconstruction. Don't get me wrong, I'm happy she's happy; I know she will feel more complete. And that's all I live for, for all my girls to feel that way.

After all, it's they who complete me.

Thanks for caring,

Mark

Back, Back and Forth

DEBBIE HAD GONE into battle, been victorious, and whatever spoils of war there were, this was the big one. New breasts. Implants to take the place of the ones removed. It was time for the payoff. Whatever silver lining you want to glean from this experience, this was about to be it, a new set of accoutrements, ones that would stick out and stand up on their own.

The downside, it meant more surgery. But this time, it was outpatient. Funny, it seemed like the surgery which removed her breasts (remember the double mastectomy) was nearly an outpatient experience, one which began a recovery process that for all intents and purposes was still ongoing. They give you more hospital time to have a baby than they do to slice off a huge part of your anatomy.

It's tough to say this was the moment we had been waiting for. It sounds contrite and cliché. And you're right. But again, if there was to be some sense of joy, besides simply being cancer free, it was to have the implants and look "normal" again, at least under garment.

And after all this, we could simply get on with life, right? Wrong again.

Gotta Give to Get: Surgery

Written September 19, 2012 12:01 a.m.

"The first time was barbaric." Leave it to Debbie not to pull any punches when it comes to words or actions. That's what makes this blog, my 50th post (figures) so easy—there's no shortage of material. As we discussed what was about to happen today, that was Deb's description of the cancer surgery, and I would have to agree. The first time left much more than a superficial scar. To say the least. The docs cut deep and so did the pain. Both physically and emotionally, the healing process will take years.

This time it's different. The understatement of our year. This time it's night and day, oil and water, sweet and sour. Couldn't be more different. Back on May 9th, the night before the surgery, I peeked in on Debbie showering with this special "surgical" lotion—given to her by the doctors as if she was sterilizing herself in advance of the "barbaric" actions to take place the next day. I lost it. Tonight, I peeked in again (I like to do that) to see her going about her normal shower routine, everything seeming to be business as usual, in our new normal.

Today, September 19th, will have a totally different feel. Not at all like May 10th, when we tried to outrun the dark cloud overhead and the quicksand underneath. Cancer was lurking in Deb's body, and the Devil was dancing at the door. Only way to beat the bitch—remove the breasts. Did it. Suffered. Recovered. Next.

We're on the cusp of Next. Today is not exactly one of celebration. No lurking surgery should be reason to get up and cheer, but it is truly the beginning of the end. The sacrifice Debbie made will pay off in the solace of a new shape, cancer free and beautiful. We have the best doctors, a great facility, incredible friends and family that lend undying support. The road to this day was not paved with gold, not even close. In fact, it was filled with roadblocks, potholes, and detours; but the Wizard is in, and while he can't bring "them" back, he can give her a solid new pair. No, not real, but spectacular.

Throughout life, you hear it is better to give than to receive. Talk about turning a phrase upside down. Deb HAD to give to get. The giving was NOT the better part. The options were few and far between. The family history made the decision, a double mastectomy, a no-brainer. I've said it before, how cancer forces sacrifice, there is just no way around it. In this case, and so many are not so blessed, we ended up cancer free and with no further treatment, just reconstruction. It doesn't end on Wednesday, but it's the last time we expect Debbie to truly go "under the knife," as they say.

Surgery 2 will begin at 11:30 a.m. today and is supposed to last about 90 minutes, then 2 hours in recovery. The muscle expanders come out, the silicone implants go in. Plenty of meds to go home with, but no drains. Can I get an Amen on that one? Recovery is supposed to take about two weeks. The pain we're told will be much, much less than the first time around. I would expect not only physically, but mentally and emotionally, as well. It's a minor surgery... all surgery is minor, until you're the person they're cutting open. Still, this time we head to the hospital, not with a feeling of dread, but with feelings of hope, anticipation, and a sense of calm that didn't exist the last time around. A new day, indeed.

At some point, and now is not the moment, I'm going to let it all out, let it all flow and write an open letter to Debbie—right in this spot and for her to keep for all time. I almost don't want to, the heart is so fragile, but it's been building for months, and I can't hold it in. Maybe Thanksgiving.

Anyway, it's a little after midnight as I click away, my bride, my hero, with her battle scars, both physical and emotional, sleeping soundly beside me. Rest easy, my love. The reward for taking such a risk is hours away. There are few who could muster such courage, perseverance, focus, vision, discipline, resilence, fortitude, and humor and have the fortune to wrap it all up in the most beautiful package I have ever seen.

You are truly the gift that never stops giving. Sophie, Emily, and I are simply lucky enough to receive. Hmmm... Maybe that's the way it really is, after all.

Thanks for caring,

Mark

Really, Really Nice...
Written September 19, 2012 1:07 p.m.

Dr. Chang came out a few minutes ago to say Debbie is all done, "They look so nice, really, really nice." He was smiling, as much as I have ever seen him smile. So am I. Much more later...

Thanks for caring,

Mark

The Twins Come Home
Written September 19, 2012 10:12 p.m.

But damn, we're exhausted. Next update, Thursday A.M. :)

Thanks for caring, Mark

Everything is Just Fine
Written September 20, 2012 6:12 a.m.

Home. It never felt so good to be back. We arrived late yesterday afternoon. I got Debbie settled in upstairs and then cracked a beer! Needed to celebrate just a little—the past 5 months have seemed like an eternity, or flew by in the blink of an eye, it just depends on the day, the memory, or your perspective. Doesn't matter at this point, it's over.

The pain is not. Deb is sore and tired. To be expected, but easy for me to say, it's not my body. She couldn't have a drink and soak in the moment of peace... not yet. Hopefully soon. There are still pain meds to take and ice to help with the swelling. But not one tear. Not my girl, she fights through it. She was the one who said to the nurse in recovery, "I want to go home." And so we did.

And here we are. The surgeon, Dr. Chang, is happy with his work. He described it as, "So so nice, really, really nice." Smiling the whole time. He should know what's good and what's not, right? He's done a ton of these. The man is a breast connoisseur. Good work, if you can get it.

Right now, a medical halter top still masks the finished product, though we took a peek last night. And Deb's too swollen and sore to start trying on sweaters just yet. :) But from the messages, texts, phone calls, and e-mails I received yesterday, there's a ton of support for Debbie's new ta-ta's.

The journey, however, is not over just yet. In a few months, there will be nipple reconstruction, tattoo, or whatever the decision is. However, it is "minor" compared to the major highway from which we just exited. The ride was one we will never forget. The destination is close.

Diagnosis. Fear. Frustration. Anger. Sadness. Sorrow. Hope. Courage. The list could keep going on and on... but we made it to this point. Deb has experienced the worst and is a survivor. A hero. My wife, best friend, and an incredible mother. Cancer couldn't change any of that, just reshape it—but she fought back to remain, at her core, the same person she has always been. What is beautiful inside shines through on the outside. Forever. You can't hold it back or keep it in. You can't cut it off or even reconstruct it. It's a gift and something you can't fake. Who would want to?

And who would want her any other way? She's simply the best.

Thanks for caring,

Mark

Guestbook Entries:

Love and light to you all! Looking forward to celebrating and toasting to those new, spectacular boobies!
Mindi Neubauer

AMEN, AMEN, AMEN!!
MY VERY BEST WISHES FOR A PAIN-LESS,
SPEEDY RECOVERY!!!
WITH SINCERITY AND HUGS,
MARILYN LEFKOWITZ

So glad this step is finished and you're doing so well. YEA, DEB! Wishing you a speedy and relatively pain-free recovery. Sending gentle hugs and all the best wishes for easier days ahead! With love and admiration,
Arlene Cohn Scherr

"I'm Over This"

Written September 22, 2012 6:39 a.m.

Even the strongest of us have our time. A crack in the armor. Deb gave in a little last night, "I'm over this," she said. I get it, but not like she does.

For more than five months, more than 21 weeks, going on half a year, she's been in pain. Not always overwhelming, but about as constant as it can be. From the day they stuck her multiple times in the breast for the MRI biopsy (April 11th) to today and beyond, she's had to suffer. The biopsy led to a huge hematoma, that was "just perfect," good work by THAT team of doctors (not our breast surgeon or plastics guy), so she had the fortune to be sore until the day they cut them off. We can all appreciate the pain following that event (or maybe most of us can't), and now the final stage of reconstruction, the implants, which have left her black and blue on both sides. Actually, purple if you want to be exact.

I fractured my fibula and was on crutches for six weeks over the summer. And, at times, I felt sorry for myself... very few times, because I only had to look next to me to put it all in perspective. My bride had a significant part of her female anatomy taken from her. I hurt my foot. Game over, set, match. It's not a competition; it's an exhibition... by Debbie in strength and fortitude.

Right now she's tired. Very tired. This isn't like the first post-surgery, but in some ways it is. Only because of the first few days of exhaustion after the "minor surgery" she went through on Wednesday. Add the soreness, bad bruising, and the emotional exhaustion of the past five months, and you have yourself quite a party.

So last night when she made the "I'm over this" comment, who can blame her. This second time around is not like some woman going in to enhance her physique. This was not a "boob job," where everything is intact. This was a replacement, for what had once been. Nowadays when the docs "pump you up" for cosmetic reasons, they cut the breast from the bottom, leaving everything the way it once was when they're done. When it's complete, the woman "pops out," but nothing has been "popped off." Debbie had her breasts "cut out" from the front, right across the middle, and that's where the implants went—same place, same scars, same pain. For Debbie's year, same shit, different day.

Don't get me wrong—they look great in shape and size, and the wounds will heal, only to have more manipulation done in two months when she makes the decision on nipples, skin reconstruction or tattoos. The finished product will hopefully make Deb feel better, physically, emotionally and—one day—be pain-free.

I almost feel bad joking about the second surgery. It was easy to view at as a simple "boob job." The implant surgery was looked upon as a minor event and really viewed as the same cosmetic enhancement that thousands of women elect to have done every year. Like her friends said from the beginning, once she was confirmed as cancer free, "She's gonna be a skinny bitch with big tits." But the statement masks the journey—Debbie can't escape how she got to this point. Neither can I.

Do I put too much thought into this? I don't care. Everybody should get to handle what happens in life the way they want, not the way others expect them to. If not for this journal, I don't know what state I would be in... and I'M NOT THE ONE WHO HAD THEIR TITS CUT OFF.

So, F*ck Cancer, F*ck Recovery, and F*ck Pain.

For some reason, my wife was chosen to go through this, and it's not as bad as it could have been, but it still sucks. Put any spin you want on it, and I've spun it around a thousand times. It still sucks when someone you love is hurting. Day after day after day. Despite her resiliency, and most who see her outside the home will never know, it's no picnic for Deb. And there's not a whole hell of a lot I can do about it, except love her. I can't massage it away, can't give her a magic pill, can't erase the hurt—outside or inside. And maybe I'm just venting, but again I don't care. It's my blog. My thoughts and our journey.

I had to walk away from this keyboard for a few minutes before I finished.

Deb is actually still asleep at 8:30 in the morning, unlike the pre-cancer Debbie, but much like the Debbie who is 3 days removed from surgery. Still, and despite my rant above, she is making great strides in only a short time. We actually went out for a few minutes last night to see our good friends, Jill and David, and visit their new home. We are fortunate enough to have them move in right up the street. We wish them only the best and are so glad they will be closer than ever. It was great to see Debbie get up and walk out of the house for a bit, and when we arrived, no one in the Suffel or Granek family could believe she was out and about, if even for a short time.

But that's Debbie. I don't sugar-coat it when I say she is the strongest woman I have ever met. How she puts other people first and, despite what she is going through, still reaches out to make sure others know that she cares. The chick is a magnet for goodwill and friendship. Seems everybody wants to be her best friend and everybody wants her involved and to be by her side. There are a billion reasons why, but it's mostly because she cares and she gives off, for lack of a better word, an aura that is intoxicating. You just want to be with her. I would know. I married her. I love her, and I just want, above all else, for her to be happy and pain-free. She'll get there, because she is stronger than I, and I have no trouble admitting it. A true hero, that's my love. And I love her a thousand times over.

Thanks for caring,

Mark

Repentance, Renewal... Nipple?

Written September 27, 2012 9:53 p.m.

A few days removed from the Day of Atonement (in the Jewish religion), a little more than a week removed from implant surgery, a few hours since our first follow-up appointment and from booking what appears will be the final "act" of the journey from breast cancer.

So how do you pay repentance during the past week of the Jewish High Holy days, when the "sin" of life was seemingly done to you? Hopefully this time around, Debbie was inscribed in the book of life for a good year... be tough to face a more challenging one. Still, hope springs eternal, right?

It was just last week that Deb had the implants inserted, and this morning we had our first post-surgery follow-up appointment with Dr. Chang's assistant. My car now automatically knows the route to Mercy hospital by heart. I said to Deb today as we approached the Mecca, "How many times have we made this drive?" Seems too many to remember. I am single-handedly keeping the valets that work the parking circle off of the unemployment line.

Anyway, I digress. The appointment went just fine. Wait a few minutes, shed the shirt, put on the gown, open it up so the doctor, or his assistant in this case (Irene), can tell us "all looks very good" and give the new "twins" a squeeze or two, just for good measure. Deb needs to start giving the new boobs a massage a few times a day to make sure the scar tissue heals okay and the implants settle in properly. Finally, I found a way I can really be useful :) Too bad she's still so sore—it doesn't do much but make her feel uncomfortable. Plus, the doctor's orders are: very limited driving, no lifting more than 5 or 10 pounds, and plenty of rest.

Yet, progress is being made. Redemption of sorts. Debbie made the statement the other day when she popped open the Velcro from the surgical halter that has become her closest friend. "They did a nice job," she proclaimed. For the first time that I can recall since last April, my bride acknowledged some beauty from the beast that tried to beat her down. It was like that first glimmer of light you see just before the sun crests the horizon in the early morning. Dawn is breaking. Debbie is peeking around the corner at the "other" side of the road ahead.

Early this afternoon, Deb made the call to Little Vinnie's Tattoo shop in Finksburg. After reading his article in the October issue of *Baltimore Magazine* and realizing he has a three-month wait to get in, it was time to schedule the appointment. We heard about Vinnie from our friends, how this Maryland guy had transformed his tattoo studio into a temple of hope, love, and jaw-dropping redemption for women forced to dance with the devil.

The guy tattoos areola and nipples—not just any nipples—3-dimensional nipples that allow his "customers" to feel like they did before. The testimonials are astonishing, gives you a lump in your throat to read them. It's inspirational. The guy is a true artist with a heart, a savior to those women who are coming to him—maybe not crushed, but previously cursed, with cancer. Vinnie is giving them a chance at renewal, a new vision for themselves, a chance to feel whole again. He's literally helping them rise from the emotional abyss.

My bride gets her shot at redemption, renewal, and a new lease on life, when we visit Vinnie in January. I'll be counting the days.

Thanks for caring,

Mark

Debbie and The O's—Miracles

Written October 9, 2012 9:39 p.m.

It was almost as if time stood still. Almost. Monday night at Oriole Park at Camden Yards, O's facing the Yankees in the playoffs. Debbie and I there together, loving and stressing over every pitch, every play, every at-bat. The place was as electric as I have ever seen it. The Orioles got the "W" in grand style. It was a night to remember, the kind of event and moment we'll tell the grandkids about some day...

And just 16 years earlier, October 1996, it was almost the same for us. Debbie and I attended the Orioles-Yankees playoff game in Baltimore that year, same ball park, different section, different result. The O's lost that one. A real heartbreaker. So much has changed; so much has stayed the same.

On that day 16 years ago, Deb and I were yet to be married, just about one month from tying the knot. Pre-nuptials, pre-single family home(s), pre-children, pre-extra responsibilities, pre-CANCER.

But there we were Monday night, together, sharing our love of just one of the things that brought us together... the Orioles. And for just a moment, as I watched the white towels being whipped around in the hands of the fans, listened to the 120-decibel cheering of the crowd, looked around at so many smiling faces, I felt like the past seven months had almost never happened. There was my beautiful bride smiling next to me, caught up in the moment, cheering with the rest of the frenzied fans, soaking in every second. No "unusual" mammograms, no needle-guided biopsies, no hand-wringing doctor appointments, no surgeries, no recoveries, no drains, no muscle expanders, no surgical bras, no pain... no nothing. Just joy.

Mark

Guestbook Entries:

I have never missed reading your posts. Unbelievable writing, Mark. Best of everything to you all and wishing you and your family a Happy and Sweet New Year.

Hugs from Debbie Foland

Mark,

You need to consider becoming a professional writer, too much talent to waste. It was wonderful to read your description of emotions and elation from Monday night; may you and Debbie share many more nights and days like that for many years to come.

Reva and Bernard

Tears

Written October 12, 2012 10:48 p.m.

"I deserved for them to win." Tears streaming from her eyes, it was tough to take, and all I could do was hug Debbie. I also felt the lump in my throat, watching the Orioles' Miracle Season come to an end as they lost to the Yankees in the playoffs. It's sad, it hurts... but YOU try sitting there while your wife completely relates what she's been through, her battle, journey and victory against breast cancer, as if the O's were playing FOR her. It was heartwarming and heartbreaking at the same time. As she wiped the tears from her eyes, I realized she had completely identified with the team... their miracle and hers. The Orioles' season is over, but for Deb it's all part of the new beginning.

I'm not so sure she was ready for more disappointment, however, especially after our high of Monday night at Camden Yards. But tonight someone was going to win, someone was going to lose. I kind of blame myself for sucking her back in this season. I was obsessed, but the Orioles were such a tremendous distraction to what we were going through, I wanted Debbie to share in the joy, as well. Unfortunately, like so much in life, joy is sometimes tempered by disappointment and sadness. Again, baseball imitating life, or is it just the opposite?

Better days ahead for all. The Orioles proved everyone wrong with a magical season that may never be duplicated. It was pure joy and admiration. The Orioles not just winning, but winning in ways that raised the bar for excitement in Baltimore sports. Debbie did just the same, showing how a cancer victim can put up a strong fight, put on a great face, and never let it stop her from being exactly the person we all love so much. You never know how you are going to react to what life hands you. Will you give up, or get up? Debbie proved to herself and everyone who knows her what she is made of. And it's pure strength, courage, and resiliency.

So this is another way to relate what happened in our family, and to the Orioles season that just completed. I didn't plan on doing anything like this last post, it just happened. When Debbie started tearing up and uttered that line... it was something I knew I wanted to document, because she had made yet another significant connection to a passion we both share. It was beautiful, meaningful, and painful all at once. It brought back the sting of loss for what she had given up, to get where she is now. I mean who wouldn't have loved to see the Orioles make it to the Series and win one for Deb, even if we were the only ones who believed that was the reason they accomplished what once seemed impossible.

So, we move on and never forget. I am sure there will be plenty more meaningful moments along the journey. Times that we will pause for a second and recognize a "connection"—times that will stay locked in our memories, be they happy or sad. A tough battle has been won, but the recovery is not yet complete.

What is complete? Two things: F*ck Cancer and F*ck the Yankees.

Thanks for caring,

Mark

I Run for You

Written October 19, 2012 10:17 p.m.

It's the weekend to Run. Really? Am I really writing about taking part in the Susan G. Komen Race for the Cure... for my wife?

How did this happen?? How is that possible?? How... do I feel?

It's not like we haven't Run before. We just did it last year. In fact, we've done it so many years, for my mother-in-law, Sharon, a 20+ year Survivor, for our friend, Bethann, a recent Survivor, for so many we know, have known, and have yet to know.

How do I feel? Does it matter? It does to me... but it's not about me; it's about Deb. So Sunday we Run for her, for the first time. Wow. Bet my girls won't complain this year how long the Run is (let's face it we do the WALK, anyway).

Not taking ANYTHING away from those we love who are Survivors, but it is different this year. The girls have already gotten a pink streak in their hair in honor of their Mom, and I just left Sophie and her friend, Asia, who were busy painting their nails pink and putting ribbons and symbols on them.

No, this year it's different.

Debbie is ready, I think. She just had her follow-up visit with Dr. Chang, the first one-on-one with him since the implant surgery. All is well, and he even gave her a RX for the nipple tattoos, which will happen in January at Little Vinnie's in

Finksburg. Bottom line is all is going well. There is still some pain and soreness, but tonight when Deb and I went out for a dinner date, she was wearing a regular bra. (But apparently not her regular glasses, she totally missed Ravens QB Joe Flacco; he walked right by us as we headed into the restaurant.) :)

Deb is ready to join the other Survivors in Hunt Valley on Sunday A.M. early... when the Survivor and Donation tent opens. There is a Parade of Pink (Survivor Recognition Walk) at 6:40 a.m. and a Survivor Photo at 7 a.m. She needs to be there... she's already said it. We all need to be there. We all want to be there to honor her because she earned it. And NEVER GAVE UP.

It wasn't so long ago that breast cancer could be a death sentence, or at least a way to be handicapped for life, for those unfortunate enough to be cursed. Now the numbers are 1-in-8 women diagnosed. But the fix keeps improving. I've said it before... it wasn't good, but it was about as good as it can get for us, from the cancer being caught early, then a brave... no, not just brave... a f*cking courageous, decisive decision by Debbie to have the breasts removed and end up cancer free. Then the second surgery and the near-perfect implants. Soup to nuts, we're talking 6 months from diagnosis to tomorrow's Race, as a walking, talking, beautiful Survivor. However, for so many, that is not the case. And that is why we still Run.

There's no cure. There's no end. But for too many it is The End. We don't just Run for those people; we grieve for them— mothers, sisters, daughters, aunts, cousins who will never see the cure. For us, those left behind, a cure can't come soon enough.

The numbers still tell the grim tale. OVER 40,000 people will die from breast cancer this year. It's still the leading cause of death for women between the ages of 40 and 55. Just because you're born a woman, you don't deserve it. No one does. It's not fair. It's heartbreaking. So we Run... to find an answer ... to find a better fix ... to find a cure. We'll never find a reason for the sacrifices that have to be made to defeat it, nor the ultimate crushing blow some families have to face when the devil gets the best of those they love the most. SO F*CK CANCER.

Debbie took her best shot and beat the beast. For her sacrifice, for her courage, tomorrow our family will Run. Because of Debbie's unwavering devotion to us, me, Sophie, Emily... even Ollie... we get to Run together. We don't have to Run away from something much more evil, which would have brought us to our knees, searching for answers that would never come. For us, it's a Run to celebrate Life.

And all we can say, and it's not close to enough, is Thank You. Thank you, Deb, for giving up to get, so we could get up... and be beside you every step of the way on Sunday... all the way to the finish line.

If anyone reading this has six minutes of your life to sacrifice, do yourself a favor, and listen to the songs linked below before the Race. The first one will give you pause, the second will bring you back... with hope! It brought Deb to tears.

(YouTube: Never Say Never Race For The Cure 2010)

(YouTube: I Run For Life- Deon Yates)

Thanks for caring,

Mark

History and the House that Love Built

Written November 3, 2012 11:30 p.m.

"And so another journey begins. However, this time it will end differently. I'll say it again—this time, there will be a different ending."

A little less than 7 months ago, that's how I began the journal entry in "My Story" on the Caringbridge website, as I chronicled Debbie's diagnosis and referenced what had happened about 2-1/2 years ago, when her dad and my father-in-law, Jerry Gross, passed away from consequences of esophageal cancer.

Today marks three years since Jerry died. November 3rd, 2009.

And I was right. There was/is a different ending. Damn different. It doesn't make the hurt from what happened three years ago any less painful, but it does prove that not all journeys have to end with a face-to-face meeting with the Almighty. With cancer, it's just how it goes; sometimes you win, sometimes you lose. Easy to write, hard to swallow.

It's a tough day for Debbie. A tough day for her sister, Alisa. A tough day for their mom, Sharon. A tough day for her Aunt Barbara. Shit, it's a tough day for all of us, for anyone who was touched by Jerry's warmth, humor, and love. Cancer took Jerry from us. Cancer took a part of Debbie with it. I've said it before, if you are so "blessed" to be in its path, you will sacrifice something, there's no doubt.

All day long, I felt like I needed to connect to the day somehow, but it was a busy one, and there was little time for reflection. In fact, it's been a busy week. Deb and I just got back from a trip to Vancouver, a work/rewards trip with my company. Even there, the subject of cancer came up again. One of our development managers was up on stage to tell the story of how stomach cancer robbed him and his three young children of his wife and their mother, at age 32. Just 32 years old. Hard to believe. His story was one for the ages... and proof of how the work I do every day makes a difference. It's all I ever want to do... make a difference.

On Thursday, November 1st, Deb celebrated her 41st birthday. Celebrate is the key word. And why not? It's been some kind of year. When we made our first toast earlier in the week, Debbie said, "Here's to a better year." You bet, and then some. What's happened is history... while the topic of breast cancer might come up, it ain't coming back.

Tonight, we spent the evening with close friends and about 800 other people at the 30th Anniversary Gala for the Ronald McDonald House of Baltimore. I am a member of the Board, and it was a special night. Hearing the stories of how the HOUSE has made such an impact on so many lives... even the lives of children who are no longer with us. It brought everything into perspective again. Just how lucky you are when your family is healthy and how lucky we were to escape and defeat the Beast this time around. So many people, so many children, are not so lucky. I wish everyone I have ever known could sit in that room tonight and hear the stories of children and families who have suffered, have come back, have lost, but all who had found respite and refuge in the House that Love Built right here in Baltimore.

There was a time, months ago, and not so far removed from her first surgery, when Debbie said she didn't want to be at the RMH Gala on the same day that marked the anniversary of her dad's passing. It was too tough a day to deal with the emotions of what goes on at the House and the painful memories of Jerry's final day. But tonight, in the middle of a speech from one of the families who had called Ronald McDonald House their home for quite some time, Debbie turned around to say she couldn't think of "a better way to honor her dad than to be here tonight." Made my heart kind of skip a beat. She got it, and she realized that we don't, we can't, live our lives in a bubble. What happens to you in your personal life might be rough, but you have to put it in perspective. So many face greater challenges, greater sorrow, greater pain. Listening to someone tell the story about the loss of their child... you understand what happened in your own life pales in comparison. And yet they find a way to go on. There should be a picture in the dictionary next to the word "Courage" for every parent who has ever lost a child. Courage, indeed.

Still, it was an uplifting evening to see those who have triumphed over obstacles many of us could never even imagine. And it actually gave a lift to what was a somber day, thinking of Jerry, thinking of Debbie's battle, thinking of how cancer has impacted our family. Thinking of how we are not alone. Not even close. We miss Jerry every day, and we cherish every moment we had with him. We celebrate Debbie every day and cherish every moment we will HAVE with her. Life goes on; our journey is not yet complete, not for a few months, but the hardship is behind us.

Driving home tonight, just a few minutes before midnight, "Til My Last Day" by Justin Moore came on the radio. I told Deb that it seems appropriate that song came along to wrap up the day, with thoughts of her dad and the stories we had just heard at the RMH Gala. If you like, search for it on YouTube.

Thanks for caring,

Mark

Moving Forward!? Not So Fast
Written November 16, 2012 6:48 p.m.

It's hard to believe. It's like someone keeps moving the flag. With the finish line in sight in just two months, the caution flag comes out. Pull over, stop, pit, and time for some repair work.

It all seemed to be going so well. Then, sometime last week, Debbie asked me if her new breasts (the implants) looked like they were "even." She thought not. I took a look—my pleasure—a good long look; they looked fine to me. If one was different than the other, it was very, very slight.

I was wrong. Almost seven months to the day since Debbie was diagnosed, she had her follow-up appointment with the breast surgeon, Dr. Friedman. The good doctor confirmed Deb's worst fears—uneven. Still, he told her she looked great. That's stating the obvious, but not what Deb needed to hear. A phone call Wednesday to the plastic surgeon's office and an appointment was set for today. We knew something was up, because they never book you so quickly.

Turns out something is "up." One of the breast implants. The complication is called Capsular Contracture. Look it up. I had to. It is defined as "a common complication of breast implant surgery, occurring in women who choose saline or silicone implants," mostly silicone, exactly the kind Debbie has. It's basically the immune system telling the body the implant is a foreign object, so in order to isolate the implant and keep it from "spreading," it creates a sac, a capsule of scar tissue, around it to seal it off. It can harden and squeeze the implant.

Ahhh. Love those scientific definitions. Give me a beaker, a test tube, and a sac around a breast implant, and I'm good all day. F*ck that.

So now it's time for Round 3. Time for yet another surgery, this time to correct the error, as we circumvent human biology and try to get things straight. Or get things even, as the case may be. It's a capsulotomy or a capsulectomy. Whatever, it's the "su" in the middle of those words that matter. Add a few letters and it spells "sucks." It sucks for Debbie, sucks for her physically, and sucks for her psyche. We were texting each other yesterday about what is going on. I told her, "I was sorry this is happening. I love you, and it will be okay in the end." Her response, "I know, I just feel really down and defeated. I don't deserve this."

You can say that again. I get what she is feeling, to have come so far, sacrificed so much, and then when you can see daylight, someone slams the blinds. I know for her what hurts the most is that the nice, perky, perfectly matching new twins were supposed to be the payoff for fighting cancer and winning. For giving up to get. To the victor go the spoils. Except war is bloody and unpredictable. Sometimes the wounds heal slowly, and patience must be treated as a true verb. Easy for me to say, or write. Tougher when you have to live with it.

So, circle December 6th on the calendar. Next procedure. Back to Mercy Hospital. Back to "sleep." Back under the knife. Back to basics. Time to correct the capsular contracture. Who comes up with these words, anyway, and why do all the things that f*ck you up seem to start with a "C"? Good thing her name ain't Charlie.

It's not fair, but in perspective, it could be worse. A lot worse. We know it. There's no chemotherapy, no radiation, not an ounce of medication needed now that cancer is history. By no means do I ever want this journal to minimize what others face with breast cancer each and every day. You are all heroes and have my ultimate respect and admiration. Forever.

Still for Deb, and us, this is a detour we weren't expecting. It's two steps forward, one step back. The silver lining... because of how quickly the next corrective surgery will take place, it should not affect the nipple tattoos scheduled for mid-January. We hope. By then, the journey will have stretched for nine months. Funny, seems like just yesterday a hole was punched in our universe. So what's another "stitch in time" to get it right and get on with life?

For Debbie, her life would like some sense of normalcy, free from doctors, surgery, and setbacks. We'll get there. You just have to believe. Sometimes that's all you've got.

Thanks for caring,

Mark

Giving Thanks: A Letter to Debbie

Written November 22, 2012 5:08 a.m.

Deb,

When they announced us into the room at our wedding on November 8, 1997, and we took to the floor for our first dance, I knew right then that my entire life had been leading me to that moment. I/we had made it to the place I belonged. It was an overwhelming sense of love, of calm, of purpose, and even as I write about now, I can still capture that same feeling in my heart.

On April 13th, 2012, when you called me on the cell phone and I heard you crying, there's that other feeling I will never forget. There was no music playing this time, no one clapping, no one taking pictures... and I didn't have the opportunity to look into your eyes and tell you I love you. There was silence for a moment, then questions ("what"?), then the obligatory, "It's going to be okay," even though I didn't know at that moment if I was really sure that was the truth.

I remember more than three years ago, the day you found out about your dad's cancer diagnosis, as I stepped back in the house after walking Ollie and saw you crying, standing in the doorway to my office, and you told me the news. Back then, it seemed more like confusion and concern about him, about hiding it from the kids for now, about what we would do for our upcoming family trip to the beach with your dad, mom, Alisa, Michael, and the girls. I won't forget that moment, nor watching him months later, slip away. It's a sense of loss that aches and stays with you the rest of your life.

So, now it was your turn. Unexpected, unfair, unf*cking believable. I never thought it would end the same way as your dad's journey, not for a moment. But I also knew the stories of what a tough, unforgiving road this could be. The uncertainty of what lie ahead and the sense of fear and sadness were palpable. I couldn't imagine that G-d was going to test us again, and this time it was my wife, partner, best friend, mother of my children, who would be forced to fight. Of all people, for someone who gives so much and is loved by so many. Wow, this sucked. Big time.

But you, scared and uncertain, to say the least, went into action, leaning on those who could make some things happen immediately. Between you, Alisa, your mom, and Lloyd... just days later, we were in the breast surgeon's office and you had made the decision to make a huge sacrifice to save yourself, but more importantly for me, Sophie, and Emily... to save us. Your decision to have the double mastectomy was swift, unwavering and so unselfish. As I think about it now, I am still in awe of your resolve to take the path. If I ever doubted you are the strongest person I know, I knew in that moment—no doubt would ever enter my mind, or my heart, again.

There were options, and you took the one that, if it worked, would give you the best chance of being free from this beast, but would leave you, for the rest of your life, with a constant reminder of what had been. It was a dramatic and defining moment for you, for everyone that knows you and loves you—and an affirmation of who you are. In our world, under our roof, in our four walls, your decision will forever be the binding force between you, me, and our girls. There is no doubt we would be lost without you... in fact, I can't even go there. But because of who you are, your resolve, and your unwavering love and devotion to your family, we don't need to think about it. Ever.

I don't need to recount every step of this journey for you; we are living it together. I can't dig down deep enough into your mind and heart to know your exact feelings. I can't live inside you, but I can exist just outside your beautiful soul. I know you have feelings of pain and loss, but I also know the other side, feelings of relief, rebirth, determination, and pride for doing what you knew was best. I don't know if joy comes into play at this moment in time—but down the road, along the better side of the journey, I know it will. As we move along the hills and valleys of our lives, there will be times, so many times for you and me, for you and the girls, for all of us together, that I hope the simple joy of just "being there" and experiencing the moments will be enough.

I can't begin to tell you how proud I am of you, of how much I love you for who you are and for what you have done for us. Your beauty, laughter, and sense of humor make every day worth it. I don't pretend to think it's perfect, every relationship, when good or bad things happen, takes work... it's all part of life and life is far from perfect, but if you have the determination to dig down deep, to never let go, and never, ever give up, it can be a beautiful ride.

So as we honor our tradition tonight at Thanksgiving and circle around the table to talk about what we are thankful for, I would never have time to express how I truly feel. Nor could I get the words out that I want to say. So I had to write it down. I had to let you know who thankful I am, how thankful Sophie and Emily are, for you. Just you. Thank you for being who you are, for giving up so much for us, for giving your heart, and your body, to make it all okay. There will never be a moment from now to eternity that we won't be in your debt. You are our hero, and we love you with all our hearts.

Thanks for continuing to make our lives as beautiful as you are.

I love you,

Mark

Guestbook Entries:

Dear Mark,

The "thank you" letter to Debbie may be the most heart-felt, genuine display of love and gratitude that I have ever read. Thank you for sharing your love story with all of us.

Debbie, thank you for being the hero for Mark to write about.

Love, Gina

Dear Debbie, Mark, and family,

We hope this Thanksgiving Day will be one of many in the future that brings each of you and your families enormous peace and happy memories. Hopefully Mark will find a publisher someday to allow the rest of the world to read his magnificent tribute to you, Debbie, a very special woman that has truly touched the hearts and souls of so many. You continue to amaze us with your strength, good luck next month.

Love, Reva and Bernard

It's like Deja Vu, All Over Again
Written December 6, 2012 4:40 a.m.

Round Three today. The first time was Fear, second was Trepidation, this time around, Frustration. But we're getting there.

It's broke, so let's fix it. Today, Debbie goes back under the knife to repair what's called the capsular contracture, basically scar tissue that has built up around one of the breast implants—the body telling itself there's a foreign invader and to stop its natural progress. In the big scheme of things, not a big deal...

but left alone, could cause pain and trouble. Besides, the "payoff" of the sacrifice of mastectomy and the reconstruction is supposed to be implants that match in size and in "location." This complication has made things a bit uneven, and medically could be a bigger problem.

So, surgery day, again. The crazy thing is it's nearly the same exact drill as the implant procedure itself, pre-op, anesthesia, surgery, recovery, waiting rooms, you know the story by now. It's outpatient, in and out. In today's world of medicine, so advanced, so cutting edge, you get what the insurance company pays for. The world's best medicine and doctors, then the McDonald's treatment... like a fast food burger, it's fix it and go. Hold the pickles, hold the lettuce. Would you like fries with that? There's no rest(ing) for the weary.

Still, this all beats the alternative, and in the end, that's the goal. Cancer came into our lives, and the doctors got it out. The rest of this is dealing with the consequences. Whatever looks good on paper, whatever plan you have in your mind, is always going to change, you have to adapt. Except, and I keep repeating this, because it's worth repeating, I'm not the one physically dealing with the pain. Emotionally, that's another matter... and for the family... not sure there's ever resolution, maybe it's simply more motivation to move on and put as much of it as you can behind you. Much like, though not nearly as intense as, death, you never get over it, you just get on with it.

And speaking of getting on with it, today's "fixer-upper" may push back the time frame for the nipple tattoos—what Debbie, for all intent and purposes, was looking to as the FINAL stage. It's scheduled for January 11th and would put Deb on track to have it all over and done with prior to Sophie's Bat Mitzvah in late March. Today's detour might mean a change to that date— possibly a big change. The doc says no, but the expert is really the "artist" who would be handling that procedure. Debbie said last night, disappointedly, that the "goal" was to have all of this done by Bat Mitzvah time. I get it. But I told her it is certainly not her fault. A goal is something you work toward with all your heart and soul, if you don't get there, you can look back at yourself, and your plan, and reflect on the reasons why. But this is not her responsibility. It is out of her control. It is much more of a milestone than a goal, a marker of time and emotion, but these circumstances have nothing to do with Debbie—and everything to do with medicine, and though I hate to say it... luck.

We are lucky. No doubt about it. Not because cancer happened, but because it's been handled with speed, with care, and with the outcome of being cancer free. Debbie has done the heavy-lifting in all of this, beginning with sacrifice. With great sacrifice comes pain, but also pride for an incredible accomplishment of will, fortitude, and freedom from the beast that tried to put a serious hurting on the future of our family. The beast defeated, the wounds are healing, however slowly.

So if the Big Three were Fear, Trepidation, and Frustration... Number Four, has to be Gratitude. Like I said, we're getting there. Or maybe, we've already arrived.

Thanks for caring,

Mark

Two for Tues... Thursday?
Written December 6, 2012 9:44 p.m.

Double your pleasure, double your fun. What we believed to be what's called a unilateral revision of the breast implants ended up being a bilateral revision. Basically repairing both implants, pulling up skin tissue here, cutting out scar tissue there, another tuck, some more stitches, a little surgical glue... it's like a field day at art class.

Bottom line, we're home, Debbie is sleeping it all off, and it's all good. Let this be the final time she has to go through another surgery. Three in a year, actually three in seven months, I think that's the hat trick. At least we hope. Each one has been a bit easier, at least from the recovery perspective. Deb already came downstairs twice since we got back, so if you're walking and you're talking, it can't be all that bad, at least from my perspective.

I got to hand it to Deb, she takes it all in stride. Though as I helped her get dressed in her groggy state in the recovery room, her exact words to me were "I'm so tired of this sh*t." That makes two of us. Exhausted is more like it. But all in all, today was more routine, or maybe we've just gotten used to the process.

The year that was, is coming to a close... though this last procedure is definitely pushing back what Debbie and I look to as the final piece of the puzzle. Even Dr. Chang admitted that the "Tats for Tits" (my words, not his) will have to be pushed back, at least two months. And now it will depend on whether the tattoo artist has a slot open that soon. He's a specialist in creating a 3-D nipple tattoo, and word has been getting around, so he's plenty busy. We'll have to wait and see tomorrow when we give him a call.

Tomorrow, by the way, is Jerry Gross's birthday. December 7th. We lost him to cancer in 2009. So Debbie's final surgery (we hope) came just one day before the anniversary of her dad's big day. I'm sure he was paying attention, and Dad, I'm sure you're pleased to know your little girl is going to be just fine. I know you wouldn't want it any other way. Miss you, big guy. Every single day.

One last thing. Before this month wraps up and before the ball drops on a new year, I'm going to ask for help from anyone who checks in here to keep up with Deb's progress, anyone who has been following her/our journey.

It's important and it won't cost you a dime, only a minute of your time. More on that in the days ahead.

Thanks for caring,

Mark

5 Hold On to My Heart

THEY SAY THAT health is wealth, and that's true. Not just in how you feel about yourself, but physically, emotionally, and financially, because cancer affects everything. It weaves its way into every part of your existence in some way, it's just crazy. And even when you think something won't be affected, it is. From the time you wake up until the time you fall asleep, you will think about it, at least once a day. Even when it's all clear.

Life after the second revision started us down a path toward a more normal existence and plenty of reflection. Soon, the more frequent doctor visits would subside, as would the pain, the physical discomfort, but emotionally, well, that's another story—a story that is still being written ... and will be for some time to come. And for THIS story, for THIS book, it was time to ask for some help.

It's Your Turn, If You'd Like to Help

Written December 9, 2012 6:06 a.m.

Not to bury the lead, but first the update:

Debbie is doing better. She's pretty sore, tired, and unfortunately had trouble sleeping. Though she's improving. Yesterday, she didn't wake until 10 a.m. The last time my wife slept until 10 in the morning was... never! And earlier in the evening, she managed to get out for a few hours and attend the Rosenfeld's Bat Mitzvah. The act falls right in line with the strength she has shown every step of the way during this journey and her constant need to give back.

So speaking of giving back, as promised this won't cost you a dime, just a minute of your time.

As we move through this month of Miracles, and whether you celebrate Christmas, Hanukkah, or Kwanzaa, it is a time for Miracles, and so I'm asking for a favor.

When I started this journal, it was for information and updates on Debbie's progress, a way to do this en masse, without calling, texting, e-mailing, or answering questions from everyone who knows and loves Debbie—and, man, let me say, there are a lot of you.

It morphed into something more, slowly and unexpectedly, a place to go to share not just the journey's progress, good or bad, but as a catharsis, to share my feelings and perceptions about what is happening. I've pretty much poured my heart and soul onto on the pages of this journal over the past year... and as you know, the journey is not yet complete. Yet, Debbie's courage in the face of adversity has made the updates almost write themselves.

But before those of you who visit here get lost in the grip of the holidays to come, I'm asking you, over the next few days and in a living tribute to Debbie, to share some thoughts on the pages of the Guestbook. There's a reason, and I'll get to it in a moment.

But what I'm asking is, if you choose, to share a thought about Debbie, whether it's a word of encouragement, a reflection, a promise of good days ahead, a story, a perception, or even sharing your own experience with the big "C." Whatever it is, it is appreciated.

Here is the reason. Come next year, I'm going to click, print, and publish this journal. Whether it becomes a keepsake for Debbie or a non-fiction book, I want you included. No one had to pay attention, but you have, and it is appreciated beyond words.

There have been nearly 8,000 visits to the Guestbook. This resonates with love and affection for what Deb has been through, how she's handled everything, and I suppose how I've documented the journey and shared my own thoughts and emotions.

So, if you wouldn't mind sharing, a moment of reflection, perception, encouragement, humor, a story, or anything you wish. You can even invite someone who might know Deb, but has never paid a visit, or someone who never met her, but simply has an experience to relate. It's all good.

During this month of Miracles, we get to celebrate one of our own, not just Debbie, but ALL OF YOU.

Thanks for caring,

Mark

Guestbook Entries:

Debbie,

I am continually amazed by your strength and courage!

I love you so much!

Allyson Simon

One of the most amazing things for me during this past year is a realization that I had. I thought I knew you inside and out. I always knew how kind, generous, hysterical, obnoxious, genuine, and sarcastic you were. But I never knew how unbelievably strong you are. You have been like a freakin' warrior! I still love you more than crab mustard and skinny cows. But after this year... I know you a little better and love you a little more (if even possible).

Jenny Schloss

Dear Debbie,

You are an example of courage, perseverance, determination, and strength. Your positive attitude has been amazing and inspiring. You are a true example to not only your girls, but to all girls. We have no doubt that your experience has impacted many women and has brought so much awareness. You have touched the hearts and souls of so many. Our thoughts and prayers have been with you every step of the way. We wish you a lifetime of good health and happiness. All the very best as this chapter closes. May the next chapter bring you and your family all that you wish for yourselves.

All our love,

Mandy, Keith, Samantha, Kayla, & Gabi Miller

Dear Mark,

Your devotion, admiration, and love for Deb are so evident in your heartfelt tribute. We all know how lucky you are to have such a kind, caring, strong, wonderful wife. That being said, she is incredibly lucky to have such a supportive, compassionate partner by her side. Your journal entries are incredibly moving and emotional. Your love for Deb is unparalleled. Thank you for continuing to inspire us through your love story. Wishing you, Deb, Sophie, and Emily peace, love, and happiness forever.

All our love,

Mandy, Keith, Samantha, Kayla, & Gabi Miller

Debbie and I have been friends since about 1985. I was lucky enough to go thru junior high, high school, and college with her. We have run in the same and in different circles over the years and have shared some unique experiences, to say the least. Debbie has been a trusted confidant, always listened without judgment, and loved me, anyway. She is, without a doubt, the FUNNIEST person I know. Fifteen years after leaving Baltimore, I still find myself laughing about something she said years ago... a face she made, a witty comeback, or the brilliant use of sarcasm she is famous for. Even our darkest days are discussed with an air of humor. I am truly a better woman, person, mother, and friend for having the gift of Debbie in my life.

Stephanie Crystal

Deb, I always smile when I see you, and you usually make me laugh, too, but just know that whenever I see you, it also reminds me of how inspired I am by your strength and grace during an extraordinarily difficult time. You're always in my thoughts and prayers. Mark, you truly have a gift for writing so beautifully and from the heart. xoxo

Lisa Sparks

Deb (and Mark, too),

You know I love you, and I cry every time I read a new post from Mark on here! I cry when he has something good to post because I am so happy for you, and I cry when there is a setback... so annoyed that you have to deal with this!! Deb, you are an AMAZING lady, which is nothing new to me, but I am proud of you every day, and here for you every day!! The whole Wachs family will always be here for you and can't wait to celebrate all good things with you in the coming months and years!! We love you!

Melissa, Kevin, Mackenzie and Spencer

The Wachs Family

Debbie,

It is very hard to describe how I felt when you told me you had breast cancer. Since our friendship began many years ago, and developed into what it is today, I have always had this overwhelming need to take care of you. When we lived together in college, I love that you depended on me to be your person and help fix things for you! When cancer was your problem, I couldn't fix it. I would have given anything to make it go away. It made me sick to think about it inside of you. I soon realized just how strong you are and that you were tougher that anyone knew! I see you now, a beautiful, healthy, strong woman... Cancer free! You look amazing and happy, and I am so grateful. While I will ALWAYS take care of you when you need me, it is so good to know that you are such a strong woman, who I greatly admire! I love you and admire you! I am so lucky to have you as my friend!

Love and Kisses, Jill Suffel

*I am thankful for my friendship with you. You are a
kind soul who is not only strong, funny, and caring, but
one of the kindest, tender-hearted, sexiest chicks I know.
I love you and am grateful every day for having you in
my life.*

Mindi Neubauer

Debbie,

*As we get ready to begin yet another year, how can I
not look back on all that has happened as we kiss 2012
goodbye? You have always been steadfast in your belief
that life is not a competition—one of the qualities I've
always admired so much in you, my dear friend. You
have always celebrated accomplishments for all and
cherished every moment celebrating life with those
you love. This year, you didn't have a choice but to
compete, and boy did you ever. I have never witnessed
such strength, poise, and determination to come out on
top. You fought hard and won big! You deserve every
wonderful thing coming your way in this new year to
come. Before me stands a beautiful friend who is healthy,
strong, and blessed in so many ways. I will always be by
your side to share the times ahead. I love you so much
and am so thankful and proud of the strong and healthy
woman you are. I am so lucky to call you my friend and
will ALWAYS be here for you!*

Love you, Lisa Carswell

How's Debbie?"

Written December 15, 2012 4:54 a.m.

"How's Debbie?" For eight months now, that's the number one
question I'm asked, and with good reason. People care, and I
am happy to share. People I see all the time, people I see on

occasion, and people I haven't seen for years... literally. Last night, I had the pleasure of attending a retirement party for "Goody," maybe one of the most respected, well-liked gentlemen to ever grace the studios of WJZ-TV with his presence. I got to see many of my former co-workers I haven't seen for years... their number one question... "How's Debbie?" "How's your wife?"

In some respects, it's why I went public with the journal. It's the ability to reach those I would never have time throughout the day to call, text, or e-mail to answer that question. And when you love someone (and there's usually a really good reason you do), you have no problem if others love her, too. Debbie has made so many deposits, either directly, or even by association, into the bank of Grace, Goodwill, and Friendship, I can understand why so many people care enough to ask.

The answer to that question is, as of today, Deb's okay. Actually, that's usually the answer I give when asked, you need to read the journal to read between the lines, sometimes Deb's better than okay, especially when she appreciates her conquest in the battle against the beast, sometimes not okay, as she deals with a consequence of that fight.

Again, my fighter gets right back up. She soldiered on and went back to work this past Thursday, one week to the day after her last surgery. Many of her co-workers, and others, couldn't believe it. In some respects, it is unbelievable; in others, it's par for the course. Debbie made the commitment to do that, by scheduling herself to work on December 13th, BEFORE she ever went back under the knife. The date carries significance, too, though I don't believe she caught onto that— it was EXACTLY eight months since the doctor called to say the biopsy was cancer... and the journey began.

Eight months and three surgeries later, Debbie was back on the job, again. She's gotten up and gotten back to work after each surgery and each recovery. It's jaw-dropping courage and commitment. As a speech pathologist for seniors at the nursing home, she exemplifies the mantra of HOPE, Helping Other People Every Day. It's what life is all about, and my girl lives it.

All I can say is Thank G-d Deb is who she is. She's the center of this family's universe. If Sophie, Emily, and I are planets, Deb is the sun; we simply rotate around her, attracted to the force, the light, and the warmth she radiates. When the center of your universe is hurting, it touches every facet of your life, emotionally, spiritually, physically, even financially. Work takes a backseat to "getting better," for everyone. I can't thank those enough who have helped out so I could still get out the door and into the office on my mission of HOPE every day, and I could never give enough credit to Debbie for doing the same. Never.

I asked a few days ago for anyone who pays attention to this journal to share a few thoughts about Debbie on the Guestbook pages (if you haven't done so already at some point). Plenty of people have; it is appreciated more than you can imagine.

Inside the four walls of my home, I appreciate with unbelievable gratitude, the abundance that already exists, with Debbie, with Sophie, with Emily, even with Ollie (our dog). I cherish every moment, and I look forward to every tomorrow.

You have to find the reason to do so... no matter what.

Thanks for caring,

Mark

Reflections

Written December 22, 2012 5:24 a.m.

They say it's the most "wonderful time of the year." These next 10 days, I think they're right. Hard not to feel that way, no matter what your religion, when, for at least a few days, or moments anyway, things seem to slow down, you take a breath, reflect, hopefully with gratitude for the good things from the past year.

Some might say Debbie and our family had a bad year. In fact, some have said it.

Bad year? Keep it in perspective. The bullets fired last Friday at Sandy Hook Elementary shot a hole into the heart and soul of anyone who is a parent. If it didn't, you need to reconsider your purpose. However, no more so than those who lost the miracle they helped bring into the world, for those who created life, having it snuffed out in a single moment, is life's greatest tragedy. Horrific. I've tried to go there in my mind; I can't because it could make you insane. How do you recover? Too many could tell their story. That's a bad year. In fact, trying to use words to describe it is just woefully inadequate.

So, perspective. Our year was challenging. Everyone has them. I elected to document this one as a reminder. At the outset, it was a way to keep the pieces of a quickly unfolding drama in order. Then as we progressed, it was a way to emote and transfer those emotions from my head and my heart into something more tangible. It has gone from a notebook of facts to a journal of observation and feelings.

Debbie. Tough choices. Tough road. Tough girl. I still like to call her a girl, makes me feel like she needs me to take care of her. (Not sure that's the case, might just be the other way around.) Tough is an understatement. From diagnosis of the breast cancer to what seemed like a snap decision of mastectomy over lumpectomy, she has never wavered and hasn't broken.

She fainted a few times, but that's par for the course. And like I said, from the outside, it might have seemed like a snap decision, but was actually a well thought out choice to pick the best chance of victory (mastectomy) over taking a stand at the front lines (lumpectomy) and possibly having to go on the attack again, because while the battle might be won, the war might not be over.

The war is over. Victory is ours. It's reason to smile. The plan was mapped out heading into battle, and while no plan withstands first attack from the enemy, in the end, the ultimate goal was accomplished. Being cancer free.

Like any war, the wounds can be slow to heal, both physically and emotionally. Scars remain and in time will fade, be covered up, or both. At least physically. Emotionally, for Deb, it's still a story unfolding.

But maybe the greatest story of the year is the one that doesn't receive the recognition it so richly deserves. Equal to Debbie's resolve, determination, and dedication to her family is all who take time to follow the journey, all who lend a hand, all who offer words of encouragement, all who say a prayer, cook a meal, send a gift, send a note, share a story, make a donation, or simply ask the question, "How's Debbie?" Friendship, concern, sympathy, empathy, and love. The heroes are all of you. We live in an abundance of gratitude because of each and every one of you. Life is not meant to be lived alone. The fortunate get to share the ride. It makes that ride meaningful, because you haven't truly lived until you have been loved by someone else. It means you have given something back to be worthy of that gift in return.

If anyone is deserving, it's my wife. Not because of the sacrifice to beat a disease, but because of the sacrifice she makes for others, her family and friends. This year, that love was returned in spades, or maybe it is every day, but it just goes unnoticed as we race through life's daily responsibilities.

But things slowed down this year. In fact, at some points, it seemed like we were moving in slow motion, and for a moment, back on April 13th, diagnosis day, time stood still. Or so it seemed. But as the seconds started ticking by again, the love and support started pouring in. Seconds, to minutes, to hours, to days, to weeks, to months of caring and concern from others. From you.

Reflection. In humans, it's the willingness to learn more about your fundamental nature, purpose, and essence. In science, it can be the return of light, as it emanates and bounces off a surface. Debbie gives off that light, and the light returned to her this past year was about as bright as I have ever witnessed. My family can't thank you enough. The journey, as it's been referred to (I guess by me more than anyone), is chapters in a much, much larger book of life. Thankfully, that book is still being written.

As we move through this most wonderful time of the year, it's a responsibility to take stock, to think back, but to do so with a focus on what went right, not what went wrong. Pay attention to the miracles and to the smallest of victories. I plan to do so, and not just this year, but moving forward. Plan for the future, but not worry about it—instead, worry about being better. What I have witnessed this past year is certainly part of the equation, and it helped lead me to a conscious decision to become MORE.

It's the attitude of gratitude that changes everything. Thanks to so many of you who helped change our lives... forever. And as always, thanks for caring.

Mark

The End of the Beginning

Written December 31, 2012 4:46 a.m.

Progress, real progress.

As we stand here on the last day of the year, I can honestly say that, for the first time in more than eight months, Debbie is feeling good, consistently good. I can tell in her actions, moods, and words. Few complaints, a positive outlook, looking forward and not looking back on what was. A corner is turned.

We talk about it some, but I get more "inside info" from the phone conversations she has with her friends. I overhear what she talks about when she describes how she is feeling and her next steps (though she would probably tell you I NEVER listen to what she says :)). We are on to the next phase. I believe she is finished recovering from her last recovery, if that makes sense. After surgery #3 on December 6th, it was yet another recovery period, the third in seven months; it's a lot to ask of anyone. But just read a few comments on the pages of the Guestbook and you see a pattern—everyone is amazed by Deb's courage, determination, perseverance, and her ability to FIGHT.

This last go-round is now nearly a month behind us and although she was much sorer than she thought she would be after the last "revision," each recovery has been just a little bit less strenuous than the prior. Or maybe we just knew what to expect and then accept. Deb still "hurts" when she lies down and tries to get comfortable, those small "heart" pillows have been a staple in our bed since last May, and she can sleep later than ever before. But she's light years from the Spring and Summer of her (our) discontent. Sleep is a good thing; when you're little, it helps you grow. When you're older, it helps you recover from your prior day of "life." Ahhh, life. It ain't always beautiful, but it's a beautiful ride.

Speaking of beautiful—2013, what will be our Best Year Ever. I've said this to several people, LIFE threw some hefty curveballs at us in this past year (we are far from alone in this). From breast cancer, and three surgeries, to a broken fibula, and recoveries (glad I could join in the fun), it was a jam-packed eight months of high spirited hi-jinks. All behind us now. Live in the present and work and look forward to a bright future.

Caught early. Contained. Stage 1. Swift Action. Surgery. All Clear.

Today, we are celebrating the end of the year for 2012 and a new beginning for 2013, cancer free and as "healthy as can be."

Yes, we are lucky. And let's keep it all in perspective. Big Time.

Last Friday night, Sophie and I volunteered at the Ronald McDonald House in Baltimore for activity time. We brought along our karaoke microphone, which we thought would be a fun holiday activity for the families. I asked the first family we met, mother, father and their three children, what brought them to the House. The father told me it was because of his 2-year-old son... who died the week before. Hard to know what to say. Hard to find words. Hard to describe what happened next.

Slowly, but surely, the families, adults and children, took to the karaoke experience. But then, the mother of the boy who had passed away decided to sing. Time stood still.

The mom, still grieving from the loss of her 2-year-old son, got up and performed a simply BEAUTIFUL rendition of Whitney Houston's song, "The Greatest Love of All." Really? Talk about courage, talk about rising from the ashes. Talk about a memory from this past year. Hadn't even talked about it yet, tough to find the words. But I and everyone there will remember it for all time.

And I'll remember every moment of this past year and never forget what Debbie did for me, for our girls, for those who follow the journey. Courage, strength, and love. It IS the end of the beginning. This past year was simply the beginning of a new life for all of us. Our Best Year Ever is here. Join us. The more, the merrier.

From deep in our hearts, we wish you a Happy New Year.

Now get off your ass and sign the Guestbook. The ball is about to fall.

Thanks for caring,

Mark

Guestbook Entries:

> *Dear Debbie and Mark,*
>
> *Thank you for sharing your story! You two are both such an inspiration, and I wish you and your family all the best in this coming new year!*
>
> *Love, Annie Ballantine*

> *Dear Debbie,*
>
> *As I reflect back on this past year and the past 11 years since Beth and I first met you and Mark, I can tell you that some of the times we spent together travelling on business trips and vacations were the best times of my life.*
>
> *You have a tremendous gift when it comes to dealing with adversity, like the time we were flying back from Jamaica in a terrible storm and the plane was worse than a roller coaster and you grabbed the flight attendant by her jacket and said, "Are we going to die?" Only you could make me laugh at a time when I truly believed we were in serious trouble.*
>
> *Your gift is your sense of humor, and I believe that is what helped you to overcome and eventually defeat the*

"Beast of 2012." You have the ability to comfort others, even when you were going through an unimaginable ordeal. This truly defines the amazing person that you are and who we love: a wonderful mother, a wonderful wife, a wonderful daughter, and a wonderful friend.

So goodbye to 2012 and let us look forward to the wonderful times we will share in 2013! We love you!

Gary & Beth Dahne

Hi Debbie,

I wanted to take a moment to let you know that I have followed your battle through Mark's journaling. I was diagnosed about a week after you were, and although my path was a bit different, (started as stage III so had chemo, surgery, now radiation), I felt we were going through this ordeal together. I have cried, smiled, and laughed while reading your story. I looked forward to the next entries and was given hope. It is amazing what we can live through. As mothers, we have no choice but to put on a brave face and maintain that positive attitude. I think the positive attitude plays a huge role in our recovery. I'm happy to know that you are cancer free. Once my treatments are over, I will finally be able to say the same about myself. Friends and family are such blessings in our lives-they give us strength through their love and prayers. Wishing you, Mark, and your girls a very healthy and happy 2013. Many blessings on all of you.

Shari Miller

For Debbie, It's a Good Read

Written January 5, 2013 6:06 a.m.

> "If you cherish a vision in your heart,
> you will realize it."
>
> - James Allen

I read this line the other day... only to realize it just happened! Debbie was sitting in bed with her iPad, (she loves that device), and as I glanced over, I saw her looking at the Caringbridge website. It was probably three days after my last post. But she wasn't looking at the most recent entry, nor was she glancing at the Guestbook, she was reading an older journal entry. Part of my vision was now reality.

It might not seem like a big deal, but consider the core reason behind all of this. When Deb was diagnosed, I made a conscious decision to document her battle against cancer, without obviously being able to predict the outcome. Knowing what this site was all about, and having seen Debbie and her sister write the updates on my father-in-law when he battled cancer—and lost—just three years earlier, it was also not an easy decision. I felt in my heart all would be okay, but in life we all know sometimes G-d tosses a curveball or two. Hell, he already had. Still, I wanted to make sure for myself, for my girls, (who don't really know about these entries), and for Debbie, there would be a way to look back and see what this is really all about.

We were lucky. There's that word again. And in the end, it's all going to be "okay." But when I saw Debbie reading a post back from the beginning of the journey, I knew in some ways we had come full circle. She was able to look back at her very personal struggle, and now has a place to go to realize just how far she's come. When you are in the heat of battle, it's easy to miss everything that's going on inside you and around you. As you move from doctor to doctor, from surgery to surgery, or from milestone to milestone, it's natural to focus only on the present and the future and forget the past. But the past is what, from time to time, should be remembered. We learn our greatest lessons from how we face and overcome adversity. But you can't just think it, you need to ink it. If someone hadn't written it down, some of history's greatest moments would be lost. The written word is worth it. Bible, anyone?

Watching Debbie take a look back at her personal history, the facts on what transpired, and my perspective on it all is truly a vision I held in my heart. I don't know if you call it a "gift" or not, but it is certainly my way of giving back to Debbie. How often will she do it? I have no idea, besides we are not yet at the finish line, if that is truly ever possible. Certainly there will be a point, probably sometime in March, if all goes well after the final stage, we might declare, at least physically, completion. We'll see. The emotional side of all of this stays with you forever; you might not get over it, but you will get on with it.

We are getting on with it, and Deb continues to show strength and a great outlook on everything. She looks great, feels good, and is even getting some garments fitted to accentuate the positive. :) Well deserved. Also well deserved, her opportunity to look back with pride on what she has accomplished, from the scary, uncertain times of last spring to every moment of triumph and setback since then. I hope she gains even more confidence, pride, and strength from reliving the journey—and how well she has handled everything. One day, I would like Sophie and Emily to sit down and read it, as well. How could it not make them even more proud and inspired by the woman they are lucky enough to call "Mommy"? I also hope and plan for this journal to be more than that—the documentation of a journey and inspiration to others who are going through the same. An emotional guide and a charitable contribution. I'm working on that. There can be a positive outcome; it's all in how you look at it, twist it, turn it, spin it, and find a way to fight through it. Find your fight and fight to overcome.

In the end, the "vision in your heart" is the key. For me, it's love. It's what gives you the fight, to have others to fight for, to be an inspiration, to give back, to be thankful for what you've got, and be thankful for others who support you and keep you moving forward. The benefits of facing true adversity change you and inspire others around you to become more. If you truly work at it, perhaps more than you ever thought possible.

Me and my girl, we're on the way.

Thanks for caring,

Mark

Rainbows

Written January 13, 2013 9:30 p.m.

Flacco's Fling and Debbie's Decision.

I started my own personal blog last week (www.markbrodinsky.com), and as soon as I hit send after the most recent post, I knew I needed to come back here for some deeper life perspective. Because the whole time I was writing it, all I could do was think of Debbie.

I wrote an entire blog post about the Raven's historic, heart-stopping victory over the Broncos and how they found a way to fight and overcome adversity, as well as answer the critics who doubted, discounted, and discouraged them, telling them there was no chance. Flacco's long bomb to Jacoby Jones was the signature play of that perfect game. It's been referred to as the Mile High Rainbow.

Couldn't help but think about Debbie and her decision back in April to take the dramatic step to fight breast cancer by taking a shot and going all in. Sometimes life mirrors the action on the field and vice-versa. Deb's choice was just like the one Flacco made. Take a dramatic step, throw the ball high into the night sky, and hope like hell it lands where you are aiming. Flacco's rainbow found a pot of gold in the hands of Jones, and he danced into football lore. Flacco was a hero.

Nine months earlier, Debbie made her own dramatic, focused, determined "deep pass" into the hands of some talented surgeons, and hoped for the best outcome. Much like the Ravens and Flacco, that Mile High Rainbow was worth it. She scored.

For the moment, lying there in recovery, hours after her long surgery, her double mastectomy, the game was tied. We were all even. The cancer had been removed, along with a major part of the girl I love. The question remained, though, would we be victorious in the end. There were still breast tissue tests to run and lymph nodes to be examined to see if any of the cancer escaped. About a week later, we had the answer. Dr. Friedman called to let us know the results—CANCER FREE.

If we had been sitting on the couch watching the whole thing play out on TV, just like we watched the Ravens game, we would have been jumping off the furniture and jumping into the air with high-fives all around. But when our big score came, Debbie was sitting there in bed, with drains coming out of both sides, pill bottles all around, and still in a good deal of pain. We could only manage some gentle hugs and tears. Still, we won; victory was ours. It was a tough physical battle at that moment and still, even at this time, takes an emotional toll.

Just tonight, as she lay there in bed, Debbie commented to me, "I want my boobs back." I asked her as nonchalantly as I could if she regretted the decision. She decisively said, "No." But I understand where her comment comes from. Who wouldn't want to truly be whole again? It's simply human nature, and it's only fair to dream.

Sometimes the rainbow, like the one Flacco tossed into the frozen Denver night sky, with just seconds to go in the game, can lead to a pot of gold. Sometimes the rainbow, like the one

Debbie launched last May, as they wheeled her back to life-altering surgery, can also get you there. It might not be a pot of gold, but something even better and more meaningful... life. I'll take that touchdown any day.

Thanks for caring,

Mark

Debbie's "Why" Power
Written January 22, 2013 9:20 p.m.

I should have known it all along, but it was so cool to hear her say it out loud.

250 days since Debbie had the surgery to remove her breasts and rid herself of cancer, we were having a conversation at a local restaurant, enjoying our date night. I asked Deb if she could do anything she wanted, what would it be? I mean was she happy doing what she does now as a speech pathologist? Does it satisfy her? Is there anything else she'd rather be doing? Debbie said "no," she loves what she does, loves helping people, loves the flexibility of her hours. All of this is important to her, because it allows her to do her most important job, the one she is commits to night and day, the one she lives for. To be a good Mom.

Man, was that great to hear. Deb basically said there is nothing in the world she'd rather be doing, because she gets the chance to do the very thing that inspires her every day, raising our girls. That's her Why.

And I know now that's the same Why that led her to what at first seemed like a snap decision to have the mastectomy, without really even considering the alternative. Yes, there was family history to consider, but that simply played into the biggest part of the courageous call—because of our girls.

Debbie never wanted to look over her shoulder again and worry that something else might happen, that the cancer could return, that it could knock her down, knock her out, or keep her from being the very thing she has always wanted to be, the very thing that gives her purpose, light, and life... being a Mom.

I'm cool with that. Who wouldn't be? While her career is important, what gives her the greatest joy in life is the thing she sometimes complains about the most, but wouldn't trade for the world, being the single most important person in this world to Sophie and Emily. Believe me, I'm not discounting my part in all of this, but I also know who my girls want when things aren't going right, and it ain't the short, handsome, bald guy typing this journal entry. Especially since the moment "you-know-what" entered our lives.

Cancer doesn't make things better, and it doesn't necessarily make families stronger. Believe me, I've heard stories where the illness can tear it all apart, in a big way. But not in this case. I know my girls respect their mom even more than they did before, though there are times I also know it's like they forgot it ever happened. That's simply a tribute to how Debbie barely allowed it to interrupt or drag down our daughters' day-to-day activities. Sure, they were sad sometimes, but never distraught. Sure, they had some bad days, thinking about their mom lying upstairs, barely able to move without pain, but their lives went on pretty much without disruption. Sure, I'll take some credit for that, but, believe me, it was because Debbie was still commanding the troops, even from her bed. Give her a phone and some friends and she can make magic happen, especially when the focus is on her girls and their well-being.

One day, not too many years from now, Sophie and Emily will look back on this time with the same unbelievable appreciation and admiration I do every day. It just simply comes with being an adult and experiencing life, lots of it, or at least enough to know when you are in the presence of something special, something bigger than you, and someone who has defined what it means to "shine." I can only hope my girls share some of the same radiance when one day they have children of their own. If the apple doesn't fall far from the tree, it will be some pretty sweet fruit, indeed.

And it's all because of the Why. Give Debbie credit for realizing her purpose, taking swift action, and staying steadfast and sure about her goal of getting better as soon as possible. To see her today, as a spectator, you would never know it happened. She is as vibrant and beautiful as ever.

Why? Because she has willed it so. Don't get in her way; her Why power is just that strong. You go, Deb, and keep on going. I love you.

Thanks for caring,

Mark

Guestbook Entry:

The other day I was eating lunch at the Brooklyn Bagel Shop, and I spotted Dr. Friedman, Debbie's breast surgeon.

I went up to him and said, "Dr. Friedman?" He said, "Yes." I said, "I am Debbie Brodinsky's mom." His reply was, "How is Debbie doing?" I immediately responded, "Very well."

After I left, I thought about that question. There is no answer that I have other than she is my true hero. Twenty-three years ago, she told me the same thing. "Mom, you are my hero." Every time the song by Bette Midler came on the radio, she would say, "Mom, our song is on." But in reality, Debbie, that song is now my song to you!!!! You are my real hero. You have shown me the true meaning.

As your parent, I only hope that I am a part of your courage and strength.

The building blocks of our family are remarkable with you making it to the top. I am truly blessed to have my beautiful daughters, granddaughters, and sons-in-law teaching me every day about life. Sometimes the blocks shake a little, but they always recover and stand tall. You are my sunshine, and I love you to the moon and back.

MOM

Cancer Free... Again

Written January 27, 2013 7:28 a.m.

The doctor comes into the room. The couple is seated across from him at his desk. He has a thick folder of test results he holds in his hands. The doctor opens the folder for a few seconds, looks at it, takes a breath and then closes it again. He says to the couple, "Look, I'm not going to beat around the bush; we've got the test results right here." Then a silent pause that is only a few seconds, but seems to last for an eternity - "You are CANCER FREE!"

Sounds like the great news Debbie and I experienced, right?

Except, in this case, we are immersed in fantasy, not reality.

So the other night, Debbie and I were watching the season finale of *Parenthood,* that NBC show based on Ron Howard's movie from some years back. The show is focused on the lives of four siblings, two brothers and two sisters. A big part of this year's show, and I have no idea why I allowed myself to get sucked into it, was focused on the wife of one of the four siblings learning she has breast cancer. Why I/we would want to relive the whole ordeal is unreal. I mean you would think we have better things to do, move on, right?

Well, we have and we do... but even I have to admit this show is a good one, and at least from our perspective, they were handling the subject just the right way. It was so good and so realistic that when the doctor announced the good news to the beleaguered couple on this fictional show, Deb and I high-fived each other right there on the couch!

The couple had been through it all. Diagnosis, disgust, fear, tears, telling the family, making some tough decisions, and in this case, chemotherapy and a lumpectomy. In fact, at one point, the wife became septic from the chemo and nearly died. She had made a video message to the family, just in case, that the husband watched by her bedside while he wondered whether she would live or pass on.

You get the point, right? So it was hard not to well up hearing those words again. So last night, I went back and looked at the journal entries I had made on "our" day, just 6 days after Debbie's double mastectomy:

May 16th, 2012:

CANCER FREE. I think next to "It's a boy" or "It's a girl" may be the two words I most wanted to hear in my life. We just got the call from Dr. Friedman, all pathology reports are in, and it's official, all clear!!

The right breast had ductal cancer and a tumor about 3mm—the left breast benign. There were two sentinel lymph nodes and one other lymph node removed, and all are clear! Dr. Friedman believes, because of the choice for double mastectomy, there may be no other treatment necessary, not even Tamoxifen. We will meet with a medical oncologist after our meeting with Dr. Friedman on June 13th. He said no rush.

What great news. What a relief. Pretty f*cking excited, if you know what I mean. I answered the phone when Friedman called, but I could tell he didn't want to tell me; he wanted to tell the patient himself. Had to wake her up for the call. :)

Debbie deserved to hear the good news firsthand. The highest peak in the journey so far. Emotions are high.

Deb, I can tell you one thing for sure: this morning's phone call was vindication of the toughest decision of your life. It was always your call, and you made the right one. How many people take that chance in life and get it right? You're awesome for your determination and your bravery. So many people love and respect you for how you have handled yourself during this very difficult time, and it only reinforces how they feel about you. Just look at the outpouring of love, cards, gifts, meals. We can never thank everyone enough for stepping up and stepping forward to help. It is overwhelming and touching beyond belief.

(End of May 16th journal entry)

Now maybe you understand why I keep the journal.

Yes, sometimes it's good to relive the ol' days, especially when those times work out in your favor.

So even on a network TV show, well-written, well-acted, expertly directed, with attention to detail (Ron Howard is still Executive Producer), the words, the emotions, the reactions are still really powerful. I don't know how, when, or if they will ever not be. That's okay. Bask in the triumphs when they happen, and rise from the ashes when you're tested. It's all part of the journey. It's why we live life, right? To be able to reflect and relive the moments, good or bad.

And not just any moments, but the moments that take your breath away.

Thanks for caring,

Mark

Nip Slip

Written February 2, 2013 7:02 a.m.

Leave it to Debbie to come up with a good one. Last night, we were attending an awards banquet for my firm, waiting for a drink at the bar, when Deb made notice of just how cold it was in the room: "It's so cold in here, if I had nipples, they would be hard as a rock right now." Nice.

Turn another corner in the journey and find humor in all that has happened, or maybe it's just the best medicine there is for healing. Either way, it's good to laugh about it sometimes... life keeps going, if you stay still, you will fall way behind.

Actually, we're not that far from what we hope will be the final physical stage of the journey. We're a little more than a month away from going to see the guy who has been proclaimed the master at tattooing the ta-tas. The work is supposed to be phenomenal. His name is Vinnie Myers, and his tattoo shop in Finksburg has become one of the best stories about breast cancer and recovery currently being written today.

This excerpt from *Baltimore Magazine* late last year: "Myers has done thousands of tattoos and works extensively with The Johns Hopkins Breast Center and The Center for Restorative Breast Surgery and St. Charles Surgical Hospital in New Orleans. Scott Sullivan, a plastic surgeon at The Center for Restorative Breast Surgery, who works with Myers, has the highest of praise. "He is the da Vinci of nipple tattoos," says Sullivan. "His work is so fine, and so detailed. I haven't seen anything like it before. His contribution to women who have had breast reconstruction is as important as anything we do as doctors."

Wow. A strong endorsement. But the real proof comes from the patients; here is one more excerpt, a testimonial from a woman who had a recent unilateral mastectomy:

"Several days after her visit to Vinnie's, she caught her own reflection in a medicine-cabinet mirror. 'The sun was coming in from behind,' Nelson recalls, 'and I looked at myself and thought, Oh my God, I'm like normal.' For Nelson, who says she 'still grieves' the loss of her breast, Myers's work has helped her heal. 'Vinnie is an artist through and through,' she says. 'He gives you everything he has as an artist and what he has in his heart.'

And Vinnie's heart, art, and talent are expanding. Finally, a quote from Vinnie himself on his website: "Many things have changed over the past few years, and now I spend most of my time tattooing nipple areola tattoos on breast cancer warriors... trying my best to get them closer to where they want to be."

Where we want to be is a little bit closer to fine. It's all I want for my warrior.

Thanks for caring,

Mark

The Shared Experience
Written February 9, 2013 6:27 a.m.

Not the first, not the last, one of millions.

25 days to go until the final physical stage of the journey. At least that's the expectation, and the recent days leading up to the Super Bowl of Survival are good ones. Debbie is living life as close to normal as you would hope. She is back to taking her Barre class and exercising almost every day, plus she's been working her tail off. My warrior exhibits strength beyond belief. She feels pretty good, has more energy (though she still enjoys a good nap now and then), and looks fantastic. All in all, I don't know how you ask for much more. It happened; it's part of your new existence, and you live and learn from it.

It's a fact that it's never far from our daily thoughts and daily we are reminded of just how prevalent the beast is, because it seems to be everywhere we turn. The problem is there are still so many stories that seem so sad. I could have sworn I heard the numbers right when we did the Komen Breast Cancer Walk back in October—if caught early, there is now a 99% survival rate. Seems like good news to me; hell, we're living a story of success. But as I've been writing a blog over at the other site (www.markbrodinsky.com) about life in general, I have been doing some research about how other people blog and the topics they choose to write about. The other day, I searched for one about cancer and breast cancer.

Sometimes a good Google search can bring you down, or maybe make you appreciate the good fortune you have. Blogs I looked at from those afflicted and their spouses had some really unhappy endings. There were good stories of survival, but still way too many of struggle and suffering. Maybe it's only when things go really wrong, people choose to share. Not here.

What it does, though, is make you appreciate and be thankful for a good outcome. Every story you see and hear, and there are millions of them, makes you realize just how many different directions the journey can take you. Some of them are directed by the doctor's decisions, some by the patient's choices, some by your mental attitude and outlook, and some... by destiny.

For us no C.R.D.—Chemo, Radiation or Drugs—made a huge difference. Boy, does that make a difference. And from what I have seen and heard from family, friends, clients, and those stories online, it is rare. Debbie's quick, but difficult, decision to go all in and do the double mastectomy had a lot to do with it, but also somewhere, somehow we were blessed. She took a huge leap of faith, and it worked out to her advantage. She certainly deserved a positive outcome, but so do countless others, and they don't always get what they deserve. It hasn't been perfect, but what war is?

Others who have lived the battle agree. I saw this post from a man who eventually lost his wife to cancer. I give him credit for his perspective, because his wife had died a month earlier, but he was still writing, creating what he said was his own personal version of a long goodbye: "It seems that people who live through wars experience the horrors of war, but also often look back on the war years fondly. I'm not sure why that is, but I think it must be, in part, because such experiences are intense, and a lot of memorable living gets packed into a little time."

I agree. And we're lucky to live in the abundance of having that time now—the time to experience what life can really be about when you stop, when you are forced to stop... but get the chance and choose to take a closer look, appreciate, dive deep into what's important, and take advantage of the incredible motivation and inspiration from the pain of adversity.

We're lucky. For us, for Deb, time marches on... and will do so for a long, long, long time to come.

Not the first, not the last, but one of millions. The journey continues.

Thanks for caring,

Mark

Heart of a Survivor

Written February 14, 2013 6:43 a.m.

This one's a layup. Valentine's Day, 2013. Easy to find meaning and gain perspective on this day. Just think, Valentine's Day, 2012, life was normal, or whatever that really means.

My bride has been through a lot since the last Valentine's Day we shared. Her heart has been scarred a bit, but it's the scars on the outside that really tell the tale of change, of courage, of cancer. The cancer is gone, but not forgotten.

We remember, but we pause today to say "I love you" to each other, to our girls, to our family, and to our friends who have stood by us every step of the way. If Valentines' Day is all about heart, this year that heart is overflowing with appreciation and gratitude for gifts of love, kindness, and caring during Deb's journey. Sometimes, the whole thing still seems surreal. Just last night, I sat with a client and friend who has known Debbie for years, and when she asked me how Deb was doing, I said "Fine." She responded, "I can't believe she (Debbie) had to go through that. I don't know if I could have done it." But Deb did it, and she's still doing it, adjusting to the new normal.

I still watch her ritual every night as she tries to get truly "comfortable" in bed. Moving around, adjusting the pillows for her head and the small "heart" pillows she holds under her armpits to keep her new breasts secure and in a comfortable position. Every night. Comfort comes and goes. But what has never left is her beautiful spirit.

Debbie has her moments, but for the most part her spirit is the same as it ever was. The beautiful spirit that refused to give up or give in under pressure. The same beautiful spirit that still has the depth to laugh, to love, and to care for so many, so many beside herself. Her drive and determination have not and will not be deterred by what cancer tried to take from her, yet I don't believe she takes much solace in her victory. I think it's more survival with an attitude and with incredible grace.

We march on now, looking forward to March and a method, still fairly new, to mask part of the outward scars of surgery. For the still healing wounds inside, there is no magic bullet, simply time. But I am certain the best medicine is to share our hearts, mine with hers, hers with mine, and ours with the girls. If time heals all wounds, then maybe enough love can make time go faster. All in good time.

On this Valentine's Day, I hope Deb feels the love, from all over, and from deep inside. First and foremost, you have to love yourself and then share that love with others. Get back what you give. My survivor is a giver and a fighter. She fought for her spirit, her heart, and to keep ours... collectively beating.

On this day of hearts, it's more than enough.

Thanks for caring,

Mark

"What About Us?"

Written February 19, 2013 8:21 p.m.

Two weeks to go. A link at the bottom of this journal entry will give you a visual on what Debbie will be doing on March 6th, as we get a shot at what you could call redemption. The last physical piece to the puzzle. Is it the last stop on the yellow brick road to Oz? We'll see.

We know this guy Vinnie does good work, or he wouldn't have been featured on a worldwide cable news network. You only make the news if it's real bad, or real good. I'm thinking he's doing it right.

I think Deb's ready... if maybe a little nervous about the "pain." She doesn't have any tattoos—I would know :), so it will be her first time. It's kind of like coming full circle in the superficial healing process, but I believe it will do wonders for what's inside, her psyche. From the stories we've read, the pictures we've seen, and the testimonials, it's all good. As good as it gets. Crazy how a little nip could make a big difference, but whatever it takes.

Speaking of crazy, it's funny how stories about the journey come out now and then, even ones you think would stay with you, but somehow you seem to forget. The other night we were out to dinner with some good friends and the topic of conversation turned to our daughters, Sophie and Emily, and how they have handled or have been affected by all that has transpired. Debbie went on to tell a story I think she only told me once, because I wasn't there when it happened.

We were at Rehoboth Beach back in August, just about eight weeks removed from the mastectomy surgery, and Debbie and the girls were wandering through one of the eclectic stores on the main strip. The topic of breast cancer came up, and Sophie asked Debbie, "What about us?" What about the chances of her and of Emily facing breast cancer? Tough question because Deb's mom, Sharon, is a survivor. The beast hadn't missed a beat passing to the next generation.

At the time, Debbie told Sophie it didn't mean that just because she, their mom, got breast cancer that they would, too. Plus, Debbie was hoping to have a test done in the fall to see if there was any genetic pre-disposition to it happening to them. Debbie recounted what happened next. Sophie told her that if it happened, she hoped it would happen to her and not Emily, because she "couldn't handle her sister getting sick." Debbie described, as they walked out of the store, how Sophie took Emily's hand in her own and they headed down the sidewalk.

Another moment. Once in a while, your kids make you insanely proud, don't they?

As it turns out, the genetic test was negative. All clear for our girls. However, the stark reality is that 1-out-of- 8 cases of breast cancer have no genetic predisposition at all. But let's not go there. Instead, let's look to the near future and our trip to the tattoo shop—where we hope dreams really do come true.

If you've got two minutes, search cnn.com: nipple tattoo artist.

Thanks for caring,

Mark

March On

Written March 1st, 2013 6:10 a.m.

The title of this journal entry says it all. Yes, it is. Yes, we will.

The first day of this new month of March brings with it the last major stop on the journey to redemption. In just a few days, Debbie will be eligible for what you could call an aesthetic stamp on this transformation from a breast cancer victim to a warrior/survivor. It's tattoo time next week.

For Deb, I hope it is part of the healing process. I hesitate to call it a "reward," it's more like an affirmation for making the right decision, for offering up a supreme sacrifice to slay the beast. Maybe it sounds too dramatic, and it's easy to look at it that way from the outside. But I'm on the inside, and even I can't ever truly know what it's like to voluntarily give up a piece of your body to save not only yourself, but the lives of others you hold so dear. Because let's face it, a different outcome would have dramatically changed our lives forever. Living and thriving would have morphed into simply surviving.

Maybe it also sounds too cliché to say I would have traded spots with Debbie in a heartbeat. But sometimes the familiar lines you hear are familiar only because if you love someone else that much, what else would you be thinking? I have a wife and two daughters, three girls who are the center of my life, and when that center cracks, or worse, a crater forms, it's my responsibility to help shore things up. Lucky for me, the woman who gave life to that center is as strong as they come.

She might bend, but she won't break. Those aren't just words anymore, either. Debbie is living proof.

So a testament to that strength comes next Wednesday, a badge of honor that just happens to come in the form of two tattoos on Debbie's breasts, a way to get back, at least in some form, what she gave up. From what I observe, other people get tattoos to send a message, to make a statement, to reinforce their feelings, or to put an indelible mark on their bodies as a way to show those they love that they will be part of them for all time. I don't have one of my own—and probably won't—but I get the point (or at least I think I do) for those who do.

The point here is the doctors say this is supposed to be the final stage of reconstruction. It's not the end of the journey, but to me, if all goes well, it's almost like walking on the moon. One small stamp for Deb, one giant leap forward for her mind, her psyche, and her heart. A chance to feel whole again.

The whole thing is just a few days away.

March on. Yes, it is. Yes, we will.

Thanks for caring,

Mark

Hard, Cold and... On Hold
Written March 6, 2013 7:14 a.m.

Good nips come to those who wait.

Apparently, that's the positive attitude we'll need to have here. Mother Nature and her late winter blast of snow have stepped directly in between Debbie and her appointment at Little Vinnie's Tattoo shop. We are in delay mode. They called yesterday to say no way for today, and rescheduled her for March 19th. For anyone who has followed this journal, or my blog at www.markbrodinsky.com, then you know how f*cking amazing it is that our new appointment is 13 days away. 13. 13. 13. At least some things in life remain consistent.

We're used to this by now. Delays in the correct diagnosis, appointments, healing, and reconstruction have been part of the journey. NO doubt they are part of any journey. So it's a few weeks more to go for physical fulfillment, at least in the aesthetic sense. In the meantime, life will go on as usual, which means expect the unexpected. Heck, if life went according to plan, we'd all be sitting around staring at each other, wondering what there was to talk about. Life comes at you in waves; you just have to ride the tide.

Surf's up.

Thanks for caring,

Mark

13, Again

Written March 13, 2013 9:27 p.m.

3/13/13. 11 months from Debbie's diagnosis today. March 13, 2013.

Time flies when you are having fun. It seems we have been through so much, yet it seems impossible to believe tomorrow we will start counting down the days to the one-year anniversary since the beast entered our lives. Fortunately for us, less than a month later, modern medicine came to the rescue, spurred by Debbie's decision to go the extra mile and make a supreme sacrifice and be cancer free.

Next week, we hope will be a very good one, as we add some color and depth to the final stages of the journey, and in doing so, cover some of the scars, at least the physical ones, that medicine, as good as it is, had to leave behind.

Debbie is doing well, looks great (I mean great!), and feels good. She still reaches for those little pink heart pillows at night to help the lingering soreness, and I think as simple emotional comfort as she handles all that the past 11 months has brought to bear. As good as science and advances in medicine have rebuilt what once was, there is no magic pill that will ever erase the memory of that time. That being said, the fear of those days has since been replaced by the fervent resiliency of a stronger woman. Stronger in mind, stronger in heart, and in incredible fortitude. Deb stands as a model to what it means to display grace and beauty under the intense pressure of a quick, fearless decision that forever changed her life. She stood her ground in the face of incredible pain and adversity. People call her a warrior, a survivor, a winner. I'm simply honored to call her my wife. I love you, Debbie.

Thanks for caring,

Mark

10,000 Times the Love
Written March 17, 2013 7:09 a.m.

This is not a numbers game. Never is. Never was. It's all about love.

But sometimes two worlds collide and you can't help but take notice, because the number is extraordinary and is a fitting tribute to the extraordinary person to whom you pay tribute by simply choosing to pay attention.

I have no idea if other people who log on to the Caringbridge site can see it, but in the upper right hand corner of the page is a ticker, a number representing how many visitors have come to read the Caringbridge page, to view the journal, Debbie's story, our journey.

Yesterday morning, that number hit 9,998. I can see it because I created the page and am the administrator of this journal for Debbie. Two visitors from 10,000. There is meaning in all of this, but before I speak to that, the story of the page and the last two visits.

When I set this page up back in April, just days after learning of Debbie's diagnosis of breast cancer, I created a campaign to allow those closest to us to view the updates, and if they so chose, to stay on top of the information as we were gathering it. This page is simply the easiest outlet to do that, rather than having to return every call, every e-mail, every text, or stop and speak to all who were sharing concern. Shortly before her mastectomy surgery, I made the page public, meaning anyone could log in, and shared the link on my social media page, because the number of people who wanted to know was growing and now it was just one-key stroke for them to stay in the loop. Going public like that took some thought, especially because I knew it meant putting this private journey under the microscope. But the support and love had already been overwhelming, so I took a chance.

I've been blown away.

Two visitors shy of 10,000 (and now over that number as of this entry this morning) who cared enough to share a few minutes of their day, especially when this journal was a nearly daily chronicle of events. The views, the comments, the guestbook filled with thoughts, support, and revelations is a complete testament to the way in which Debbie lives her life—always giving back, always being there for others, always, even more than she knew herself, being strong.

Two visitors away from 10,000. The number means nothing and means everything. I decided at 9,998 it needed to mean more, so I made a decision. I wanted those two visitors to be two people who are at the very core of this very personal journey, yet barely even know about the existence of the web page, Sophie and Emily. My daughters know the website exists. I've mentioned it in passing, but we don't say more about it than that. Neither Deb nor I believe there is any reason for them to be on this site. They have lived the experience, and it is up to us to filter the information to them, especially in the darker days last spring and summer.

But the story has turned out okay, and on top of that, I really felt I wanted them to be part of, what I guess, would be best referred to as another moment in the journey. So I decided this one time it was worth orchestrating history, because in the not so distant future, in the pages of a book, I want them to take part. I instructed each of them how to go to the Caringbridge website, to create a log in and then log on to their mom's page. First Sophie, 9,999. Emily, 10,000. Then unsolicited, they each posted a one-line message to their mother on the guestbook page.

"I love you, Mommy."

It's just a number. I know it. Yet, even as I write about it at this moment, that "moment" made my eyes fill with tears. Because I know it's those two people, our daughters, for whom Debbie's decision has the greatest impact, now and forever. Her choice to take the life-altering chance to rid herself of cancer, in essence, made their lives complete. Because without her in their lives... well, it's really not even worth thinking about.

But this I will think about. You. The other 9,998 visitors. And I can't even begin to describe what it means to know that so many care, and so often, and want to share. Your love, support, and the attention you pay to this journey is overwhelming. Hard to believe even I can't find the words, though I know it's not really about words, it's about the return on an investment.

The investment Debbie has made in her life to be that special person to whom so many others respond.

It's your response that has changed our lives, and, make no mistake, it is changed in ways we are only beginning to understand. I can't say this with enough conviction to show you how much we truly appreciate, admire, and are forever grateful for all that you have done and continue to do. Your simple awareness and attention is love in its truest form.

I can only say what I always do and know that I mean it from the very depths of my soul...

Thanks for caring,

Mark

Guestbook Entries:

I love you mommy - Sophie Brodinsky

I love u mommy - Emily Brodinsky

Coup De"Ta-Ta"? Not Even Close

Written March 19, 2013 8:25 p.m.

When my girls were very little, one of their favorite bedtime stories was a book by Nigel McMullen called *It's Too Soon*, about a young rabbit who keeps complaining that it's too early to go to sleep. Today, Little Vinnie wrote the adult sequel and turned out the lights.

I'll make a long story short, so you don't fall asleep. Picture this: Debbie back in the "surgical" room at Little Vinnie's Tattoo Shop, her top off, covering herself only by holding a paper gown up to her chest. Vinnie had already written down all her breast cancer information and left the room, while Deb undressed, leaving me, Debbie, some heightened anticipation, and a little anxiety for what was to come next.

Vinnie came back through the curtain, sat down, rolled his chair closer to Deb, and she lowered the paper gown. He said her scars looked "fresh," then he reached for some cleansing wash and started to rub her breasts, I assumed to wash them off before getting started.

I was wrong.

He suddenly stopped rubbing. "It's too soon," he said. "I can't do this; it wouldn't be right." Vinnie said the scars on Deb's breasts from her most recent revision back in December were still healing. He couldn't place a nipple areola or tattoo there, because it would only have to be fixed again later. If he did create the tattoos now, the scars would heal more and create a white line right through the artwork—and it would not look good. That was all Deb really needed to hear. I could see it in her face, and in her eyes, she didn't want to hear any more, but Vinnie kept going. He was drawing on her breasts now and showing her where he would have created the nipple tattoo and why he was concerned. But Debbie wasn't really listening; I could tell she was already done; she just wanted to leave. It wasn't happening today. No how. No way.

"Disappointed" is what Debbie said a few minutes later, as she slowly got dressed. I knew, and I could see, that it went deeper than that... for both of us. Today was supposed to be another milestone, another marker along the journey, and one that represented a real mental and emotional signature, a chance for Debbie to look and feel "whole" again. But it was not to be, not yet. It was a slap in the face. But after getting punched in the stomach about a year ago, when we first learned of the diagnosis, a slap is not quite as bad.

Still, imagine running a marathon, and with just a few feet to go before you reach the end, somebody jumps you from behind and pulls you to the ground, holding you down. You can still see the finish line, almost touch it, but the person holding you back is not allowing you to budge an inch. You're stuck. And then you're told you can cross over, but not today, it's going to be quite some time, you'll have to wait. The new record time you had hoped to get is long gone... and now it will only be in time, much later in time, that you will get to finish the race.

That's where we are. We're now looking at September 4th, 2013 as the new target. Vinnie said six months would be a good measure of time to get everything healed to the point he would want to move forward. I credit Little Vinnie for stepping up big, by pulling back. He told us some others might have done it, but it wasn't going to be him. He is doing us a huge favor and doing the right thing, but it still stings. Physically, outwardly, no one can tell a thing. It's not like if Debbie got the nipple tattoos she was going to run around pulling her top off and showing the world. It's not what this is about, never was. It's about the mental and emotional resurrection and some rebirth for what the cancer killed off. Deb has been in a funk all day, and I can't blame her.

A disclaimer, because there is more to the story and it bears sharing. We know we're "lucky" in terms of survival from breast cancer. It could be much, much, much, much worse. We hear the stories and we have lived them—losing Deb's dad, Jerry, a little more than three years ago to esophageal cancer. It took only six months from diagnosis of cancer, to surgery, to complications, to death. And all through her own ordeal, Deb has barely shed a tear. Because she knows "life" is the ultimate prize. Still, like Deb said tonight, once in a while she knows it might not be right, but she can have her own pity party. She's only human.

So here's the silver lining, the takeaway from what was taken away today. Vinnie told us both that Debbie is an incredible story. She represents less than 1% of the people he sees. For her to go from diagnosis, to surgery, to being cancer free, to implants, to revision to be standing here in his studio—in less than one year—is phenomenal. He might not have been able to give her a tattoo or two today, but she has been given much more, a story of survival that is the envy of so many others. Vinnie told us the woman who had the appointment just before ours was 37 years old and has had 13 surgeries on one breast. (There's that number again.) It's hard to imagine.

It certainly puts it in perspective, which Debbie and I have no shortage of these days. But, when you live it, sometimes there are those moments when even though you know you're fortunate, you yearn for just a little bit more, a payback for the sacrifice. Maybe someone to throw their arm around you and say, "You know what, it's okay. You did it, so here's a small gift for doing such a great job and for being so strong."

Yes, today was to be much more than just a tattoo. Still, we didn't leave empty handed, or empty hearted. We left with another moment in time that only brings us closer, a moment we will look back on one day and remember how it made us stronger, and made us realize just how lucky we are.

Little does my wife realize, or maybe she does, that I already have a tattoo. It's sits deep inside, stamped on the confines of my heart.

The tattoo has a name... Debbie.

Thanks for caring,

Mark

Guestbook Entry:

Mark & Debbie,

When I read your updates, I realize the distinction in life between what is important and what is "bullshit." We may be worried about the drive to work, will we have time to get to the grocery store, what will happen at work, etc. Then we read about the incredible journey your family has been on, and everything falls LOUDLY into perspective. We are all lucky to be alive! It's the first day of spring, and today I will try to express and feel gratitude because your journey and your journal have put things into focus. Debbie will get her nipples, but the next few months will seem so long, and I am sorry for the wait, it doesn't seem fair... Thanks for sharing the details, another prayer going up for your family right now, and Vinnie made the right call. (Can't you get some stickers or some other "temporary" nips?) This will be on my mind today. All the other stuff we fret about, it's bullshit. What you guys have been through, that's real-life and brutal.

Brenda Carl

Her Purpose... To Party

Written March 26, 2013 9:24 p.m.

Back in April of 2012, our thoughts were far from the details of a special celebration, but not that far. My daughter Sophie's Bat Mitzvah was to be held this month, March 2013, less than a year from diagnosis of breast cancer, and although survival was the ultimate goal, Debbie never lost sight of the time period, when if things went right, she wanted to be healed. She was going to dance at her daughter's Bat Mitzvah on March

23rd, 2013. She was going to be recovered, be ready. And in nothing short of a miracle, she was.

Over on the pages of my personal blog, www.markbrodinsky. com (In Full Bloom & Don't Stop Believing), I re-capped how it all played out this weekend for us and for Debbie. It was something else, because my wife is something else.

Debbie had her hand in every detail of the weekend's festivities, from a pre-party dinner on Friday, to the big day, to a brunch at our home the day after. All of this, despite the fact she had her hands full for much of the year, just trying to stay on her feet. From May through December, there were three surgeries... the first of which was a life-changing double mastectomy. From recovery, to recovery, to recovery, Debbie never lost sight of the big picture for Sophie's big day, and she never stopped planning. In some ways, I believe it was cathartic for her. It gave her a diversion from the pain, as she focused on piecing together the puzzle pieces of an event this big. It was living proof that if you have a dream bigger than you and you put your heart and hard work into it, you can overcome almost any obstacle.

While I managed her meds, Deb was manager of her manual with all the details of the party... from contracts with the party place, to people handling the decorations, to a photographer, a videographer, the DJ and dancers, the party favors for the kids, the tutor for Sophie, the guest list, the invitations, the table seating, the dresses, the makeup, the list goes on and on. I never heard Deb complain. And I didn't do much to help. She had it under control. My job was to complete the video montage for Sophie and to get a suit. And just in case you think my wife simply sat around and planned a party, she certainly did, in between working her job as a speech pathologist 2-3 days a week. Oh, and had I mentioned the rest and recovery, the rest and recovery, the rest and recovery...

So as she stood there Saturday night with Sophie, Emily, and myself at the front of this huge room and welcomed the 200+

who we (she) invited to attend the celebration, Deb was about as radiant as could be. And with good reason. It was hard for me to hold it together when it came time to talk about Debbie and her success at planning this major milestone in our lives. I had to push back my emotions, so as to give her the props for fulfilling what became her purpose this past year. Sophie's Bat Mitzvah gave Deb focus and a goal to go for, and she arrived, healthy and more beautiful than ever, if that is even possible. Everyone in the room that night knew her story and many have devoted their time to reading and following our journey. I know they couldn't help but admire the same woman I am blessed to call my wife.

And that was why, about four months before the big day, I decided I needed to pay tribute to Debbie at that party, by telling her in song just how I felt, along with a video montage which included pictures and words that described Deb and her battle—words like strength, beauty, courage, warrior, survivor. The song I chose was "I Won't Give Up" by Jason Mraz, and the lyrics vow to keep looking up, even when the skies are rough, and to keep on loving because she is worth it.

I know I'm still looking up, at someone who has done more than most people could have imagined this past year. With her sacrifice, fight, and focus, she made her little girl's dream, really all of our dreams, come true.

Thanks for caring,

Mark

And Then There Were 10

May 1st, 2013 6:00 a.m.

Ten days.

A lot transpires in the course of anyone's life, and inside the nearly 365 days since diagnosis, it seems like an entire lifetime has happened. The journey that began on Friday the 13th of last year continues today.

Though our big moment will come on May 10th, the one year anniversary of being cancer free, I would like to pause to say this to all of you who have taken the time to follow the story. If love is the world's strongest emotion and "I love you" its power phrase, then a close second are the words "Thank You." Thank you from the very depths of our hearts for being there, each and every day, for showing you care, for your support, encouragement, and your participation in the relief and celebration of being cancer free.

They say no dream is possible without a team; thanks for joining ours. You can't imagine how family and friendship have helped immensely in every step since the battle began. The journey has been enriched by the lives of those who have chosen to touch ours. In life, health is wealth, but it is also defined by the relationships you develop and the lives you touch and that touch yours along the way. Thank you for choosing to touch ours in a way we will never forget; you are forever in our hearts.

Ten days. We're almost there.

Thanks for caring,

Mark

Guestbook Entries:

I think about how few "man" hours I have actually logged with Debbie. I don't see her nearly enough, and our friendship is relatively new compared to others she knows... but the feeling I get when I am around her is hard to describe. She makes me smile just from the look in her eye. Before her mouth opens, I am laughing because I know something ridiculous is going to come out. It's funny how just a quick thought about Debbie makes me feel lighter. Usually, I walk away from her thinking, "How can I be more like that?" I guess that sums up how I feel about Debbie. I wanna be more like her:), minus all that cancer crap. XOXO

Jenn Stevens

I never go on this because I talk to you every day, so I figure I can say things to you then. But while we are so busy talking about how many peach rings we consumed, or I'm being immature and doing endless stupid impressions, I guess I forget to mention that you blew me away with this whole "cancer thing." The fact that you are so immature like me made it so shocking to watch you beat cancer like the most grown up strong woman I have ever met! From the second you called me to tell me you had cancer, you had this tone in your voice—you calmed my nerves and fears. You were so worried about me and so sure of your plan. I knew, during that phone call, that you would be fine. You have been nothing but a pillar of strength through this whole thing. But thankfully you can still be obnoxious with me. I know I turn to you often and say, "I cannot freakin believe you had cancer." I guess what I really mean is I cannot believe how you kicked cancer's ass!!! My goofy ass best friend handled it like a soldier, and I thank g-d every day for that!!

Jenny Schloss

May 9, 2013 9:09 p.m.

Well, Debbie... I don't have a way with words, and it doesn't come easy for me to express myself for everyone to read! I must really love you! How you once were this shy little girl who couldn't look you in the eye to the strongest little fighter I know blows my mind!!! I admire everything about you. I've shared some wonderful memories with you for 35+ years, and I want to continue!! You did good, kid, I love you with all my heart!

Andi Resnick

You are a remarkable family, thanks for sharing your journey. It has been a privilege to be a part of it.

Love to all of you,

Jan Silhavy

It Takes 2

6 A DAY TO STAND FOR ALL TIME

IT'S ONLY ONE journal entry. But it deserves its own chapter, because in all that had come before, it closes the book on a part of the journey. One Year Cancer- Free. Just writing the words brings elation, celebration, some trepidation (still), and tears. It evokes pride, confidence, and concern for the emotional journey which truly has no end, but has reached a high-water mark. The chapter doesn't need a long introduction, it speaks for itself. The title of the journal entry, I had kept locked inside my head, ready to display, ready to remember, ready to honor my hero.

CFD is a BFD: One Year Cancer Free

Written May 10, 2013 4:11 a.m.

Sometimes the title says it all. CFD is a BFD. (One Year) Cancer-Free Day is a Big F-ing Deal. Maybe all the years will be big. Moving forward, there will be anniversaries, but it's only the first year you can look back on and let out that sigh of relief... because THIS is the year IT happened.

I didn't buy a card for the occasion. I didn't buy flowers. I didn't buy a bottle of wine. But I do have a gift, so here it goes.

Dear Debbie,

Five Hundred Twenty-Five Thousand Six Hundred Minutes. How do you measure a year in a life? I'm about to tell you.

The past year has been one we won't soon forget. Today, one year ago, you were preparing for a life-changing surgery, which you faced with determination and strength. I still remember the nurse taking your vital signs and then saying, "You're a perfectly healthy 40-year-old woman, except you have breast cancer." I can still see them wheeling you down the hallway, away from me, toward the operating room, knowing it would be the last time I would see you exactly the same way, and it had nothing to do with how you would look coming out.

No, it had everything to do with the person I saw in recovery—the woman, who at that moment, became a hero to all who love her and to all who know anything about her. Debbie, you acted swiftly and without hesitation to make sure you would be the same person to us... to me, to Sophie, to Emily. You made a huge sacrifice, and because of your will to give of yourself, we got more than the person who had just hours before sat shivering in a hospital gown, about to face one of the biggest moments of her life. In return, we received a stronger, more resilient, tougher, and even more beautiful person, inside and out, if that's even possible. Now you were a warrior, a survivor.

And make no mistake, beating breast cancer had nothing to do with you and everything to do with you. The doctors stepped in for the surgery, and the results were positive, in our favor, big time. They took control, and we lucked out. But when the last stitch was sewn, the last drain removed, the final pill popped, at that moment, the medical book closed. The next story to be written was up to you. Where do you go from there?

I'll tell you where, and it's not down any yellow brick road. You got up, you got out, and you got on with it. Debbie, you showed our family, you showed everyone, how it's done. Our lives, mine, Sophie and Emily's, barely skipped a beat. How is that possible? It seems impossible; yet ordinary people do extraordinary things all the time. It was only possible because the person who took the punch got right back up and carried on. Deb, I don't know what we would do without you. You continue to amaze me and your girls every single day. You gave up so much and yet were able to still give so much in return. You exemplify what is right about life; those who face adversity can truly become more than they ever were before. You had every right to go the other way... breast cancer is a bitch. So unfair. It's a shame that you, or any woman, should have to suffer, just because what makes you different can, without warning, be ravaged by bad cells. The very thing that physically makes you female, suddenly makes you sick or worse, can kill you. It's a f*ing crime.

But there were few tears here. Plenty of tired days and nights. Plenty of pain and physical suffering. But you, my love, kept most of it out of sight. Instead, you put on the brave face and showed the sense of humor which endears you to so many. And, G-d forbid, you could ever let what happened cause you to skip even a step from being there for whatever your girls needed. You stayed steadfast and on course with life's most important responsibility. Sophie and Emily are who they are because of you, and believe me, they have learned so much, even if they don't show it yet. How could they not? Their mom is one of a kind.

So it's time to celebrate, to celebrate life and how it continues to be this crazy ride. One Year Cancer Free—the words sound good to say, good to hear, and as good as it gets. And on the cusp of another Mother's Day Weekend, I simply want to say thank you. I think I've done a fairly good job over the past year of making sure my words would be something we would remember. My words had power, especially for me, because without the chance to write, to share our story, and to let my feelings pour from my heart and onto these pages, I'm not sure what I would have done.

But sometimes words fall short. And this is one of those times. I could write for days, months, or years and never be able to truly express how I feel about you and what you mean to my life. I might not always say it, either, but I can only hope from this past year, from my posts, from my actions, you are beginning to get the point.

We go back a long way. I've known you since you were in your teens. I fell in love with you when you were in your twenties. I've admired you for what seems like a hundred years. And I will respect and love you for all eternity.

One Year Cancer Free. Here we are.

Thanks for caring,

Mark

Afterword
The Summer of 2013

The surgeries and recoveries of the summer of our discontent in 2012 are but a whisper in our memory. Or maybe I'm the one who hears the whisper, or chooses to, anyway. For Debbie, the sound is a bit stronger, after all, it was her breasts that were removed and she lives every day with the replacements, not me. Still, I would like to think even she hears the sound of the cancer drum beating only in the distance, removed from her body, though never far from her memory.

What's the takeaway in all of this, in battling breast cancer, even in what I would call the "best of circumstances?" It's that from the time I heard the word "cancer" until the day we celebrated the one-year anniversary of being cancer free, I never could truly catch my breath. I could breathe in and out, but not deeply. My heart is still recovering from the beating, mostly from my **reliving** nearly every moment through this journal. It was my choice, my catharsis, but by reaching deep into myself and viewing my wife through that same lens, I stretched my heart to its limits, released it, stretched it again. Day after day, month after month. So in that respect, my heart has grown. It's bruised, it's battered, but it's bigger. I can feel more deeply, love more deeply, experience life more deeply than ever before. Debbie gave up her breasts, but I believe we both have found a higher purpose, in ourselves and in each other.

The physical journey will take us back to the tattoo shop in September. At that point, maybe, just maybe, the looks in the mirror for my bride will become a bit easier. I hold out hope in the testimonials of those who have received the nipple tattoos and have been reborn, or at least been brought back to a place in their hearts and in their minds, to feel a sense of completion. It's all I want for Debbie. It's all I ever want for Debbie. To feel the same way she makes my life ... whole.

Thanks for caring,

Mark

(Get updates on the journey, access to support groups, resources and cancer-related organizations at the official website for It Takes 2, www.spouses-story.com. There you can share a story, give feedback, comment and view the special book video trailer!)

Debbie's Message

When Mark asked me if I wanted to express any thoughts or feelings about this book, I was truly at a loss for words. This experience has been life changing in many ways. It has opened my eyes to what is important and what really matters in life to me. I read through these journal entries, and I feel like I am reading about someone else's life—that somehow "this" didn't really happen to me. But it did, and I feel so fortunate to be where I am now. I am healthy and happier than ever. I would like to thank everyone for their love and continued support, mostly, to my husband, Mark, whose love is the definition of unconditional. I love you and am so grateful to you.

It Takes 2. It truly does.

Xoxo

Debbie

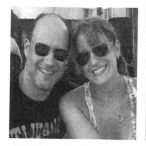

Everybody wants to meet a *hero*. I'm lucky, I'm married to one.

She makes me proud to be her husband.

My wife continues to *amaze* me every day.

The most satisfying moments in life are the ones you *struggle* to achieve.

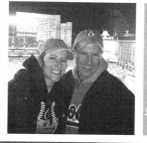

I will see you on the other side of the surgery, *my survivor*

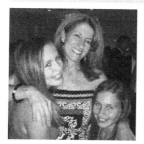

Cancer forces sacrifice.

Cancer is like *dancing with the Devil.*

I just *wish* I could take the pain away for her.

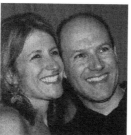

I've been humbled.

You are my motivation, my inspiration, my hope, my world and *my very best friend.*

We are forever in your *debt.*

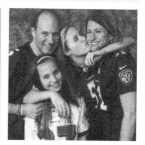

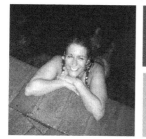

Five Hundred Twenty-Five Thousand Six-Hundred Minutes.

To feel the same way she makes my life... *whole.*

I Love You.

About Mark Brodinsky

Mark Brodinsky is the husband of a breast cancer survivor. For more than a year, he kept an emotional journal of his wife's battle with breast cancer, describing Debbie's journey through his eyes and through his heart. Mark took their very private journey and made it public on the pages of Caringbridge.org and Facebook and thousands responded.

Mark "The Blade" Brodinsky, as he was known at WJZ-TV in Baltimore, is an Emmy-Award winning TV producer and on-air talent. He has worked for more than a dozen years in the financial services industry, selling millions in health and life insurance. Mark publishes a daily Wordpress blog, *It's Just About... Life,* (www.markbrodinsky.com), where he shares stories of inspiration, motivation, gratitude, and simple observations of life and love.

Mark and Debbie are the parents of two girls, a teen and a tween, Sophie and Emily. They currently reside in Owings Mills, Maryland.

Mark welcomes your comments and feedback, and he invites you to share your own story by visiting his website, www.spouses-story.com, or send an e-mail to markbrodinsky@spouses-story.com.

Portions of the proceeds of sales of *It Takes 2* will be donated to several cancer-related charities and organizations, including Caringbridge.org.

26516615R00107

Made in the USA
Lexington, KY
05 October 2013